CONSCIOUSNESS:
How the Mind Arises from the Brain

Stephen Goldberg, M.D.
Professor Emeritus
University of Miami School of Medicine

Made in the United States of America

Published by
MedMaster, Inc.
P.O. Box 640028
Miami, FL 33164

ISBN# 0-940780–74-7

In memory of Zak

Other MedMaster titles by Stephen Goldberg:
Clinical Neuroanatomy Made Ridiculously Simple
Clinical Anatomy Made Ridiculously Simple
Clinical Biochemistry Made Ridiculously Simple
Clinical Physiology Made Ridiculously Simple
Ophthalmology Made Ridiculously Simple
The Four-Minute Neurologic Exam
Goldberg's Brain Model
Neurologic Localization (Mac/Win)
Jonah: The Anatomy of the Soul
The Jonah Principle: The Basis for Human and Machine Consciousness
Consciousness, Information, and Meaning: The Origin of the Mind

TABLE OF CONTENTS

PREFACE

The Mind/Body problem, a long-time subject of philosophical and scientific discussion, is the question of how conscious experience can arise from the brain. We smell a rose, but where is the rose in the brain? I have written this book with the idea that there is still something more to be said. I propose a different approach to the problem.

One reason for confusion in the field is the language that authors commonly use. While specific jargon often arises in a field to facilitate communication, it sometimes gets in the way, particularly when different authors define the jargon differently. Indeed, sometimes debate centers not around whether or not a particular author is correct, but around what the particular author actually said. I have tried in this book to present the issues with a minimum of jargon for greater clarity. I have not sought to deliver an encyclopedic review of the literature, since excellent reviews already exist (e.g., Dennett, '91; Chalmers, '96; Blackmore, '04). Rather, this book focuses on a particular idea as to how to resolve the Mind/Body problem.

I first define what I mean by consciousness and indicate why the Mind/Body problem is important. I then present thoughts toward a solution. Although I have taught the anatomy of the nervous system for some 25 years, only a small amount of neuroanatomical detail appears in this book, because I feel that what is really needed to resolve this issue is a change in our customary concepts of space, time, and reality. The point of view that I have expressed is that consciousness has a far more universal existence and is not just confined to the brain.

I thank Ron Fisher and Phyllis Goldenberg for many helpful comments.

CHAPTER 1. THE DEFINITION OF CONSCIOUSNESS AND THE MIND/BODY PROBLEM

By consciousness I mean the experience of the color "red," the taste of "coffee," the smell of "rose," the sound of "C sharp," the feeling of "pinprick," the emotions of "fear," "anger," "hate," and "love," the thoughts that continually run through one's mind while awake or dreaming.

By consciousness, then, I refer to the actual feeling (referred to technically as "qualia" in the literature) of "red," "coffee taste," etc., as opposed to the underlying neuronal circuitry in the brain. This book is about the singular issue of trying to understand how consciousness can arise in the brain (and elsewhere).

The problem of consciousness has been divided into the "easy" problem and the "hard" problem (Chalmers, '96). The "easy" problem (not actually so easy) is trying to find the neural correlates of consciousness, i.e., trying to discover what neural activity is going on in the areas of the brain associated with consciousness. Regardless of what physical activity occurs in the brain during consciousness, the question still arises as to why those goings-on should give rise (or correspond) to consciousness. The language of the "easy" problem is that of neuroanatomy, neurophysiology and neurobiochemistry. There will be little discussion of these subjects in this book, since the focus of attention is not on the easy problem, but on the "hard" problem. The "hard" problem is why the brain, regardless of what its neuroanatomy, physiology, or biochemistry might be, should give rise to the qualitative experience of consciousness. Why should there be any consciousness at all? It would seem that we could just as well have the same anatomy, physiology, and biochemistry, but without the consciousness. Why are we not just zombies? (The term "zombies" in philosophical discussions does not refer to dead bodies that arise from the grave to terrorize the village, but to the prospect of a human acting in a perfectly functional manner, but without the experience of consciousness.)

Evidence points to the brain as a source of our conscious experiences:

- Nerve pathways from the sense organs in the eye, ear, nose, tongue, and skin trace to corresponding areas in the brain, which, when stimulated with electrodes, can duplicate the conscious experience. Imaging studies, such as the

PET scan, light up specific areas of the brain in correspondence with particular conscious experiences.
- Destroying those key areas of the brain can erase the ability to report corresponding conscious experiences.

Yet the conscious experiences themselves do not resemble the neuronal structure that is associated with them. We do not find the conscious experience on dissecting the brain or contemplating its neuronal circuitry. How does consciousness arise?

In this book, I will use many terms synonymously with "consciousness," such as "qualia," "awareness," "experience," and "mind," and even, toward the end of the book, "soul." I recognize that there are subtle differences in the meanings and usages of these terms, including that of the word "consciousness" itself, but it may help here to skip the subtleties of language and focus solely on the "hard" problem.

It is important to be clear about the usage of the term "consciousness," since a large problem in the literature has been the different definitions assigned by different authors, leading to confusion in communication and authors talking past one another.

To the neurologist "consciousness" refers to a clinical state. The "unconscious" patient in neurology is one whose mental function has so deteriorated that the patient becomes nonresponsive to deep pain stimuli.

In the philosophical literature, some authors define "consciousness" as "consciousness of self." I do not use the latter definition, which is a rather high level of consciousness. Much lower levels must be considered as well. In my usage, a person or animal may be conscious of red, but not necessarily conscious of his/her self at the same time. A cockroach running from danger may have a very low level of consciousness of some sort, for instance, without having consciousness of self.

Some authors define "consciousness" as "consciousness of consciousness." That is, they consider consciousness to be an awareness that one is conscious. Again, I do not use the term in that sense. For instance, today I was conscious of enjoying breakfast but never once thought that I was aware of being conscious of this. I was still conscious of breakfast, though. My dachshund, Zak, responded with a yelp when his tail was accidentally stepped upon. He may well have been conscious of pain without experiencing consciousness of self, or consciousness of consciousness.

"Consciousness of self" and "consciousness of consciousness" are treated in this book as special complex types of consciousness, which need separate explanations in themselves but are not necessary requirements for consciousness per se to exist.

Thus, the particular definition of consciousness and the Mind/Body problem that I employ is a rather simple one, that of the experience itself, as opposed to the brain tissue, where the experience seems to arise. It is not a question of whether this definition of consciousness is correct. It is a semantic issue, one of personal choice, rather than one of correctness, as to which definition to use. I find that this simpler definition will avoid much confusion in trying to understand consciousness, whether at the simpler or more complex levels.

CHAPTER 2. THE IMPORTANCE OF THE MIND/BODY PROBLEM

The Mind/Body problem is a series of related questions:

- How does consciousness arise, or is it a pseudoproblem, only "seeming" to be real? If it is a pseudoproblem, how does our brain trick us into thinking that there is such a thing as consciousness?
- At what level of biological (or other) complexity does consciousness arise? Or does consciousness exist at all levels of complexity?
- When did consciousness arise in evolution, or has it always (or never) existed?
- Does consciousness have a use? Could a zombie, a hypothetical being that acts like a normal person yet has no consciousness, be just as functional? Can there be such a thing as a zombie?
- What accounts for consciousness of self?
- What accounts for consciousness of consciousness?
- What accounts for the binding of consciousness? That is, a multitude of neuronal events in our brain at different locations and times occur during a given conscious experience. Why do they appear bound into a single conscious experience, rather than separated into fragmented bits of consciousness?
- Why is the consciousness of one person not bound to the consciousness of another? Or is it?
- What makes certain areas of the brain "conscious" and others "nonconscious"? Or are all areas conscious—or nonconscious?
- Are nonhuman life forms conscious? Are inanimate objects conscious? Is there a consciousness to Nature, to the Universe as a whole? Is there a Mind of the Universe, which one might refer to as "God"?
- Is there such a thing as "free will"? If so, how could this arise in the brain?

Why should anyone be concerned about these issues?

- The topic of consciousness partly relates to the legal system, where we consider the individual to have free will and behavioral responsibility in committing a crime. Hence, does free will exist or is it but an illusion in a deterministic universe?

- Questions about consciousness have religious relevance, not only as to the question of free will, but also to the question of the existence of God: What does the concept of God as the "Mind of the Universe" mean in relation to the question of the nature of the human mind? Can one learn something about the meaning of what is referred to as "God" by understanding the nature of human consciousness? Is there a consciousness that exists at a higher level of complexity than that of humans? Or are minds, whether that of people or God, an illusion? Is there such a thing as a "Soul?" If souls exist, are they any different from minds?
- Evolution has built into the human psyche the strong need for survival. Is there a consciousness after death, or do all vestiges of the human mind disappear with death? We would like to believe that death is not the end, but is it?
- It is intrinsic human nature to inquire into the deepest workings of the universe. Consciousness is a mystery that intrigues people, as do the mysteries of the origin and evolution of the universe, and the fundamental propositions of mathematics and physics. There is great interest in the relationship between consciousness and quantum mechanics, relativity, and theories of the origin of the universe. What are these relationships, and are they valid?

Hence, there are good reasons for examining the subject of consciousness. In this book, I hope to provide some insights into the nature and origin of consciousness, focusing exclusively on the "hard" problem. As mentioned, there will not be much neuroanatomy in this book, since, despite my teaching the subject for 25 years at the University of Miami School of Medicine, it is my view that neuroanatomy, neurophysiology, and biochemistry in themselves do not suffice to help us understand the hard problem. Regardless of what the neuronal circuits are, there still would remain the question as to why they should give rise to consciousness. Unraveling the mystery of consciousness requires a different approach.

CHAPTER 3. THE ORIGIN OF CONSCIOUSNESS—CURRENT THEORIES

In a broad sense, there are two major theories of consciousness: the dualistic and monistic approaches.

The *dualistic approach* proposes that there are two entities, the mind (consciousness; qualia) and the brain. In this view, events in the brain somehow give rise to consciousness in a mystical mind outside the brain, and the reverse occurs as well: the mind may communicate with the brain to take action. The difficulty with this approach, though, is that there is no known physical mechanism that would enable events in the brain to transform themselves into the conscious experience. And there are no known receptors in the brain to receive any messages from a conscious mind.

The *monistic approach* proposes that only one entity exists. This view may be divided into either *monistic materialism* or *monistic idealism.*

Monistic Materialism

In *monistic materialism,* there is no mind; only the objects of the world exist. The brain and its activity alone suffice to account for what we call human conscious experience, which may well be a pseudoproblem, in which consciousness only appears to exist but really doesn't. The advantage of this approach is its simplicity in not requiring the introduction of the mysterious entity of Mind. The disadvantage, though, is its denial of the very thing with which we are most familiar (arguably the *only* thing with which we are familiar), namely conscious experience itself. It is difficult to accept that consciousness does not exist and that we are fooled into thinking that it does. To the materialist, consciousness is a pseudoproblem, in which we only "seem" to think that we are conscious, and all that really exists is the brain and its physical activity. It is difficult, though, to accept that "red," "taste of coffee," and "pain" are not real experiences.

There are many examples in psychology where the brain deludes itself. For instance, when a picture is presented in a certain perspective, the reader may think that one object is larger than another, while both are really the same size. However, in this example, everyone would agree that the observer actually experiences one object as larger than the other. In the case of "taste of coffee," there should similarly be no doubt that the observer actually experiences the "taste of coffee." The observer doesn't just "seem" to have the experience. The experience is there. One would have to account for why the observer has, or feels that she has that particular experience. It is hard to reject the existence of the feeling itself, the *experience* of sight, sound, taste, smell, touch, emotions, and thought.

The following thought experiment, though, seemingly provides a reason for favoring monistic materialism:

> Imagine a nonconscious (zombie) computer that has the ability to compare inputs and report whether they are similar or different. For instance, in **Fig. 3–1** the computer is first presented with the sound of a car horn (call this Event 1).

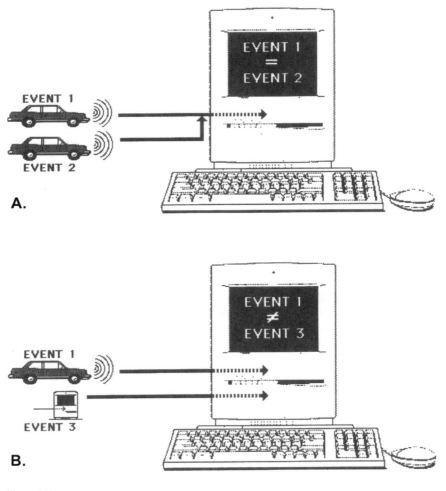

Figure 3-1

Sound detectors register the sound and code information about it in a form that is stored in a region in the computer's inner circuitry, in which only sound data are registered. From our perspective, the only thing occurring in the computer is activity in certain electronic circuits. There is no consciousness.

Now the sound is played a second time (call this Event 2). This time, the same circuits fire. Assume that the computer has a mechanism that allows it to detect whether the same area in its circuits has been fired a second time. The computer then concludes that Event 1 is the same as Event 2. The computer flashes on its monitor "Event 1 = Event 2."

Now imagine (Event 3) that the computer is presented the second time not with the sound again but with a picture of all the flashing spatiotemporal patterns in its electronic circuits that were firing when the sound was first played. One can present this information to the computer in any variety of ways, e.g., a moving picture of the circuits firing in which transmitted messages are outlined in color; a mathematical printout of sequential electronic changes of state at various points in a large electronic network map; etc. It may be difficult to present all this information to the computer, but let us take the liberty to assume it in principle. We thus present the computer with the circuitry picture of Event 3, a picture of itself in the act of "thinking," which it detects through special light sensors; it relays these data to areas in its circuitry that record light data. We now ask the computer whether Event 1 is the same as Event 3. No matter how we present the spatiotemporal pattern of information to the computer in Event 3, it is going to activate areas of the computer's circuits that *differ* from the areas that were activated when Event 1 occurred. The computer is geared to detecting whether the circuits that fire during two events are the same or different. The computer must therefore conclude "Event 1 is not equal to Event 3." That is, the experience of Event 1 (the "sound") is not the same as the experience of Event 3 (the circuits that fire during registering of the "sound"), so the two must be different.

The computer seems to be saying that the "sound" it experiences is not the same thing as the data processing in its circuits during the processing of the sound input. The computer is describing a sort of dualism when none actually exists.

Let us now consider the same experiment in a person (**Fig. 3–2**). We ask the person "Is Event 1, the sound, the same as Event 3, the data processing in the brain," or, more briefly, "Is this (play the sound, Event 1) the same as this (show a moving picture of the circuits of the brain firing, Event 3)?" The person will answer "No, they are different. One is the sound of a car horn. The other is a picture of the brain, which is quite different from the sound itself. I have a Mind, which experiences the sound, and I have a Brain, which may be necessary for me to experience the sound, and which fires as in Event 3 when the sound is played, but the Brain is different from the Mind." Unknown to him, we are simultaneously monitoring all the activity in his brain while he is evaluating and responding to our question. We find that his brain, as does the computer, compares the two events. The circuits that fire in response to the car horn differ from the circuits that fire on presentation of the picture of the spatiotemporal patterns of car horn neuronal firing.

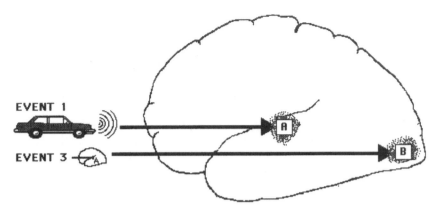

Figure 3-2

This leads the person to conclude, as does the computer, that Event 1 and Event 3 are different and to tell us this. *Even if the person were a zombie and the only thing that happened was the firing of circuits, and there were no such thing as consciousness, the person would still tell the experimenter that the sound and the circuits are different and that he (the subject) has a "Mind" and a "Brain"!*

Now this is a most peculiar situation. Here we can show that even if there were no such thing as the experience of consciousness, the person may still report "consciousness." Do we then say that consciousness does not exist, that the whole issue is a pseudoproblem in which the brain is tricked into thinking that there is something called "consciousness?"

The problem with this reasoning is that it is still not so easy to dismiss the issue of consciousness as a pseudoproblem, because what the person reports is not just a "difference" between his original input and his visualization of the events that occur in the brain during the input processing. The person specifically reports, "I see 'green,' I feel a 'pinprick,' 'I smell a rose,' 'I taste coffee,' 'I hear the sound'." How does one account for the actual color, pain, smell, taste, sound, etc.? These are much more specific than just a "difference" between the original input and the visualization of the circuits acting during the input. Where do these specific experiences come from?

Monistic Idealism

Monistic idealism is the opposite kind of monistic approach. It assumes that only consciousness is real, that the physical world is an illusion. It has the advantage of avoiding the issue of how the brain gives rise to consciousness, since the only thing that actually exists in idealism is consciousness itself, and consciousness rather than the "real world" is the only thing we ever experience. The disadvantage of this viewpoint is that it is hard to deny some degree of reality to the outside world and the physical brain itself. If there were no reality to the outside

8

world or brain, how would we be able to survive and communicate with others, or have a concurrent agreement about what an outside world looks like? Or are there no other people, and there is only one consciousness (mine? yours?), the *solipsist* point of view, where everything results from the hallucinations of one mind (in which case there would be no point in writing this book, trying to convey ideas to others, who do not exist). Or perhaps there is an outside world, but it, too, consists of consciousness (an idea to be explored toward the end of this book). While monistic idealism attempts to resolve the hard problem by eliminating the question of how the mind arises from matter (there is no matter, only mind) it substitutes a new problem, namely, "How does matter arise from mind?"

CHAPTER 4.   TOWARD A NEW THEORY OF CONSCIOUSNESS

I will attempt a solution to the Mind/Body problem through three proposals:

Proposal 1: *Consciousness is information.*
Proposal 2: *Consciousness comes in a broad spectrum, from very simple to very complex.*
Proposal 3: *All areas of the brain are conscious.*

Proposal 1: *Consciousness is information.* Equating our consciousness with the information in our brains provides a ready approach to the Mind/Body problem. This is a dualistic formulation that does not require a mystical supernatural Mind. However, proposing that our consciousness is the information in our brains leads to three immediate questions:

- If consciousness is information, and information can be complex or simple, does this mean that consciousness can be ascribed to even simple levels of information processing?
- There are many areas of the nervous system that engage in complex information processing, but are not believed to be conscious. If consciousness is information, how would one then account for the (supposed) unconsciousness of these areas?
- What is "information"?

The first two questions are addressed in Proposals 2 and 3. The third is the subject of much of the book.

Proposal 2: *Consciousness comes in a broad spectrum, from very simple to very complex.* Thus, even a cockroach, as it flees from a threat, has some measure of consciousness. This does not mean that the roach is thinking "I better get away from that person before I get stepped on." It may have a much simpler form of consciousness that is too elementary for us to appreciate because higher elements of consciousness (e.g., consciousness of self) are such a staple part of our own consciousness whenever we think of something.

I propose that consciousness comes in even very simple forms, because if we assume that consciousness requires a certain degree of complexity before it arises, we then have great difficulty explaining why consciousness should suddenly arise at a particular point of complexity. That is, why would consciousness not exist when 1 billion neurons fire but suddenly arise when 1 billion and one neurons fire? The nature of consciousness differs so radically from the physical nature of neurons that it is difficult to explain why it should suddenly arise at a certain level of complexity. If a fetus only becomes conscious at a certain stage of development, what was its status one minute before that time?

We can see, for instance, how a home, which differs from a brick, can arise from a pattern of bricks. Both the home and bricks are in the same category, that of the physical. But it is difficult to see how consciousness per se can suddenly arise from a particular complex pattern of nerve cell firing, but not exist with a pattern of lesser complexity. Why should consciousness, a category so different from matter, arise with just a higher degree of complexity? There may be different degrees of consciousness associated with different levels of complexity, but why should consciousness per se be totally absent at one level of complexity and suddenly pop into being at a higher level? It is more reasonable to consider consciousness as a continuum, becoming more complex as the complexity of its underlying physical substrate increases. I propose, therefore, that consciousness exists all the way down to the very simplest of levels.

Scholars often claim that consciousness did not arise in evolution until the nervous system achieved a certain level of complexity, as if there were no consciousness at all below that level of complexity, none for the initial billions of years of cosmic evolution. In part, this claim is an example of ambiguity in the definition of consciousness. If by consciousness, one means the human variety of consciousness with the full gamut of self-consciousness and consciousness of self and higher order thoughts, then of course consciousness as so defined would require a certain high level of complexity to exist. Consciousness would not exist in other animals if the bar of complexity is raised high enough. It would not have existed at an early stage of evolution but would have had to wait until the development of an advanced type of primate. The problem with this reasoning is its all-or-none claim that there should be a sudden ushering in of consciousness per se when complexity reached a certain level, and that there is no consciousness at all before that level is reached. Why should consciousness suddenly arise at a certain stage of complexity?

As another way of looking at this problem, imagine someone saying that the concept of "city" emerges from the idea of a number of houses or other buildings clustered together, but then states that the idea of "house" has no subdivisions from which the concept of "house" emerges. That would be preposterous, because "house" consists of subdivisions (of walls, roof, windows, etc.). The concept of "walls" emerges from still lower subdivisions, of wood planks, plaster, and so on to lower and lower levels of molecular organization. How could one say that there is emergence of city from houses, but there is no emergence of "house" from anything? Yet there are theories that propose that there was no consciousness at all in evolution until a certain level of complexity was achieved. One would have to explain why a certain level of complexity arrived at through evolution should be accompanied by consciousness, but not lower levels of complexity. It makes more sense to think of consciousness as a continuum from elementary to complex.

Proposal 3: *All areas of the brain are conscious.* There are no unconscious areas. This proposal at first may seem absurd. It seems so "obvious" that certain areas of the brain are associated with consciousness, while others are not. For instance, if one stimulates certain areas of the cerebral cortex (the layer of neurons on the surface of the main bulk of the brain, the *cerebrum*), the subject will report a variety of conscious experiences, e.g., visual or auditory hallucinations, depending on the area stimulated. But stimulating the *cerebellum,* a smaller structure which lies below the cerebrum, does not give rise to the report of a conscious experience. This has led to the assumption that the cerebellum is not a conscious area of the brain. Such logic is flawed, however, for the following reason:

Imagine that there is a very advanced whale that is not only conscious but also able to describe to others what it is conscious of. The whale swallows Jonah, who is also a conscious being. Despite the fact that Jonah resides inside the whale, the whale is not aware of Jonah's thoughts. If one asked the whale whether or not it was conscious of Jonah's thoughts, the whale would say "No." Should one then conclude that Jonah was not conscious? Of course not! Just because the whale was unaware of Jonah's thoughts does not mean that Jonah is not conscious. Jonah is just unable to communicate his thoughts to the whale, but he is still a fully conscious entity, and a rather complex one as well.

Now let us return to considering the cerebrum and cerebellum of the brain. When the cerebellum, the so-called unconscious area of the brain, is stimulated, the person does not report any conscious experience. Does this mean the cerebellum is an unconscious area of the brain? It is unjustified to conclude this, just as it is unjustified to conclude that Jonah in the whale is unconscious. The cerebellum may be perfectly conscious, like a Jonah-in-the-whale (perhaps to a more elementary extent) but just unable to communicate this to the person, so the person cannot report being conscious of the cerebellar stimulation. We hastily conclude that the cerebellum is unconscious, whereas it may well be a "Jonah-in-the-whale." *I refer to the latter type of hidden, but real, consciousness as a "Jonah-mind," as distinguished from our "customary" consciousness, the latter being the kind we customarily experience and can report on in our daily lives.*

Both the Jonah-mind type of consciousness and our customary consciousness could be similar except for the nonreportability of the Jonah-mind. Jonah cannot report his consciousness to the whale. The reason the whale cannot report its consciousness of Jonah's thoughts has nothing to do with any lack of memory or with complexity of the thought process. Jonah has no difficulty with his memory and his thoughts may be quite complex. The problem is one of communicating his thoughts to the whale. He could have a mind just as complex and just as capable of memory storage as the whale, but this would not suffice to enable the whale to be aware of his thoughts.

A Jonah-mind does not have to be as complex as our customary consciousness. It need not have consciousness of self, or consciousness of consciousness, or other features of higher levels of customary consciousness. But even if it did, the person still could not report to others about the Jonah-mind's experience (any more than the person could report on what someone else was thinking), so it remains inaccessible to customary consciousness, while nonetheless remaining conscious in its own right. In principle, a Jonah-mind could be quite complex or quite simple. I use the term Jonah-mind to affix in the reader's mind the idea of a *hidden consciousness,* rather than our customary consciousness that we can readily report to others. Just because the name "Jonah" is used, this should not lead the reader to think that it necessarily refers to a little person, or homunculus, in the brain with the consciousness of self or other higher aspects of consciousness. A Jonah-mind may be quite elementary, referring conceivably even to the information inherent in just two neurons that are in association. A Jonah-mind may be simple or complex.

Disney's Epcot Center contains an exhibit called "Cranium Command," in which a person takes control inside the brain of a 12-year-old boy. The stomach, cardiac, and endocrine systems are presented humorously as separate people, who have their own thought processes and report them to the pilot in the control system in the brain. I do not have this in mind in describing Jonah-mind type consciousness in so-called "nonconscious" brain areas. In Cranium Command, the pilot (the brain) is conscious of the thoughts of the other people (the organ systems), who report to him. In contrast, a Jonah-mind does not communicate its thought processes to the person (except perhaps for the final results of the thought process, e.g., nausea, as opposed to the underlying physiologic events that give rise to nausea). A normal person will state that he is not conscious of the detailed thoughts stemming from such a purported Jonah-mind. Moreover, the organ systems in Cranium Command are portrayed as individual complex people, but a Jonah-mind does not require complex customary consciousness. It does not necessarily have a concept of self, and the qualia that it experiences do not have to be complex.

Why postulate the existence of the Jonah-mind? Without this assumption, we are left with the dilemma as to why one area of the brain should appear to be conscious and another not. All areas of the brain are complex. Why should consciousness be associated with one area and not another? Some researchers have proposed that there are physical differences between one brain area and another that may account for their being "conscious" or "nonconscious," such as 40 cycle/sec neuronal electrical activity confined to the "conscious" areas (Crick, '94; Blakeslee, '92, '95), or complex thalamocortical neuronal circuitry associated with consciousness (Edelman et al., '00). However, these proposals do not explain why a physical difference of any kind should result in one brain area being conscious and another not. This difficulty disappears with the Jonah-mind, where it is proposed that all brain areas are conscious. It may simply be that some areas can report to the outside world on their consciousness while others cannot. The difference between the conscious and so-called "nonconscious" areas is the same difference that accounts for why the whale is not aware of Jonah's thoughts. It has nothing to do with complexity. A Jonah-mind can be highly complex (like Jonah-in-the-whale) or simple, with no advanced features like consciousness of consciousness, or consciousness of self. The difference may have to do with reportability, not complexity. The problem of understanding why one area of the brain and not another should be conscious then disappears. All areas of the brain would be conscious, but some would be conscious in the customary sense, others in the Jonah sense.

In addition to explaining the supposed discrepancy between "conscious" and "nonconscious" brain area, the assumption that all areas of the brain are conscious is necessary to be able to propose that consciousness is information. Since there is information everywhere in the brain, it can be equivalent to consciousness only if consciousness is everywhere, too.

The proposals in this book, then are:

- *Consciousness is information.*
- *Consciousness may range from simple to complex.*
- *All brain areas are conscious—the Jonah-mind.*

These proposals will be used to develop an approach to resolving the "hard" problem of consciousness, namely how consciousness actually arises in the brain.

It will first be necessary to define "information."

CHAPTER 5.   CONSCIOUSNESS =
INFORMATION = MEANING

If we define consciousness as "information," we need to be clear about the meaning of "information," a word that has more than one usage in the literature.

In information theory, which is not the subject of this book, the term "information" is used in a much different sense than its ordinary usage. "Information" in information theory refers to the minimal number of binary digits necessary to transfer a message, and does not take into account the *meaning* of the information. This technical use of the term "information" is quantitative rather than qualitative. It is sort of like describing the difference between an elephant and a car in terms of their weights. That may be important if one is trying to determine the weight capacity of a ship that is trying to carry an elephant or a car. However, it does not tell you anything about the actual difference between an elephant and a car. Information theory concerns itself with the most efficient way to transmit data, using the fewest binary digits. The "meaning" of the data is another matter. As Weaver points out (Shannon and Weaver, '63):

"The word *information,* in this [information] theory, is used in a special sense that must not be confused with its ordinary usage. In particular, *information* must not be confused with *meaning.* In fact, two messages, one of which is heavily loaded with meaning and the other of which is pure nonsense, can be exactly equivalent, from the present viewpoint, as regards information. It is this, undoubtedly, what Shannon [a pioneer in the development of information theory] means when he says that 'the semantic aspects of communication are irrelevant to the engineering aspects.'"

A picture of a house and a picture of a car might contain the same quantitative measure of information in information theory, requiring the same number of bits to transfer the message of either picture from one place to another. Nonetheless, the information in the two pictures is considerably different in the qualitative sense of "meaning."

Conversely, two shaded circles may look identical and have the same meaning, but be much different in terms of the measure of information, as assessed in information theory. The one shaded circle, for instance, may be constructed using a computer "vector" draw program, and require very few bits of memory to store the information, because it is drawn using a mathematical algorithm for constructing a shaded circle. The other circle, while appearing identical, may require many more bits of information to store as a "bitmap" image, which records the exact pixel location of each shaded point in the circle.

As Pierce observes in regard to the differences in usages of the term "information":

> "It is natural to say that both men and horses run . . . and convenient to say that a motor runs and to speak of a run in a stocking or a run on a bank. . . . It would be foolish to seek some elegant, simple, and useful scientific theory of running which would embrace runs of salmon and runs in hose. It would be equally foolish to try to embrace in one theory all the . . . sorts of [definitions of] communication and information which . . . philosophers have discovered." (Pierce, John R., '80)

I suggest in this book that consciousness is equivalent to information. Information here, though, refers to the more common usage of the term "information," namely the qualitative usage, which is "meaning." It is that qualitative definition of information which I believe is most relevant to understanding consciousness

But what do we "mean" by "meaning"? I do not refer to "meaning" in the mystical sense of purpose as in the "meaning of life" or "meaning of the universe." I refer to a rather simple usage of the term, that of *what the object or activity refers to*. For instance, a word can have a meaning, sometimes more than one. The sound "hee," for instance means "he" in English, but means "she" in Hebrew. The sound "dog" refers to the canine species in English but means "fish" in Hebrew. "Hee" actually has an infinite number of meanings in respect to an infinite number of yet unknown interstellar languages, all defining the sound differently.

A code, e.g., a computer code in C++, has a meaning in regard to the translation key that it refers to. The circuitry code for a circle in a computer becomes translated into a picture of a circle when transmitted to the computer screen and in that overall context has the meaning of the picture of a circle. Without the connection between the computer and the environment (computer screen in this case), the same code could have numerous meanings in respect to an infinite number of translating systems. If the same circuits with the "circle" code, for instance, were connected to a speaker, it might have the meaning of a particular sound, rather than a picture. Similarly, an isolated music CD does not intrinsically contain the information that says "sound." If the CD were connected to a visual screen, it could just as well contain the information for patterns of light.

Similarly, the human brain, like the computer, has a code in the form of its particular pattern of circuit firing. I use the term "code" in a very broad sense, implying not just the rigid type of digital code found in the typical serial-type processor of current computers, where precise directions are carried out one at a time (serially, one after the other). Code directions could also be fuzzy and approximate, and operate in a parallel processor, such as the brain, where each neuron acts as a miniature computer unto itself, contributing directions in synchrony with many other neurons acting in parallel.

But if information in the brain is in coded format, what establishes the meaning of that code? The reality of the outside world does not reside in the brain. That is, when contemplating a tree, there is no tree in the brain, but there is a representation of "tree" in some sort of coded format. Where is the translator for that code, the dictionary that provides meaning to the neuronal firing patterns in the brain? This is an important issue, to be elaborated upon in this book.

If consciousness = information = meaning, then it resolves the key objections to both the dualistic and monistic approaches. As the meaning inherent in the firing of neurons, consciousness is not a mystic force outside the brain located in a strange dimension. Rather, it is of necessity inherent in the activity of the brain. It is the *meaning* associated with the activity in the brain.

If our customary conscious experience is the "meaning" associated with the firing of nerve circuits in the brain, how does that meaning arise, and how does the person know about that meaning? Where is the translator that gives rise to that meaning? I hope to systematically work through these issues in this book.

CHAPTER 6. FORMATS, CARRIERS, AND TRIGGERS OF INFORMATION

In order to further clarify what is meant by "information," it may help to point out entities that are commonly confused with "information" when discussing activities in the brain. These terms are *"Formats* of information," *"Carriers* of information," and *"Triggers* of information."

Formats of Information

It is important to distinguish information from the *format* of the information. Information can often be represented in more than one format. A piece of music that is represented as a series of waves on a tape can also be represented as a binary code on a compact disc, or as notations in a musical score on paper. We say that the information on the tape is the same as that on the compact disc and sheet music since, in the presence of the appropriate translator, one format can be converted to the other and to similar-sounding music. Two objects may contain the same information but exist in different formats. *The format is not the information.*

Carriers of Information

It is important to distinguish information from the *carrier* of the information. For instance, the plastic/aluminum structure of the compact disc *carries* the music information but is not *the* information. The magnetic tape of the tape recorder carries the music information but is not *the* information. The tape, the compact disc, and the paper carrying the musical notation carry similar information but are different carriers. Thus, information may remain the same even though the carrier of the information may change. *The carrier is not the information.* The brain is the carrier of the information of our customary consciousness, but the brain itself is not the information.

Triggers of Information

It is also important to distinguish information from what is a *trigger* of information. For instance, imagine an arrow that flies through the air, striking a particular point of the visual area of the brain, which when stimulated will give rise to the visual hallucination of a specific scenic landscape. The arrow does not contain the information for the landscape but simply *triggers* the brain into calling forth the landscape image. A pinprick that elicits the sensation of pain does not contain the information of pain. If the same pinprick were applied to the retina, the experience would be that of a flash of light rather than pain. Nor does a "red" wavelength contain the information of "red." It could just as well contain the information for "heat" when striking the skin as a laser beam. *A trigger is not the same as the information that arises in the brain in response to the trigger.*

Thus, in order to understand what "information" means, we should *avoid confusing information with formats of information, carriers of information, and triggers of information.*

CHAPTER 7.   INTRINSIC VERSUS EXTRINSIC MEANING IN CONSCIOUSNESS

The proposal in this book is that consciousness = information = meaning. Using "meaning" as a synonym for consciousness does not help, though, unless we can clarify still further what is "meant" by "meaning."

The term "meaning" is used here to signify what is represented or implied by a symbol, what the symbol refers to. A meaning may be *intrinsic* or *extrinsic*. For instance, a circle, on the one hand, is the set of all points equidistant from a single point on a two-dimensional surface, which, when created, forms a path that has no beginning or end. That is the intrinsic meaning of a circle. These qualities of a circle would be recognized by anyone from a distant planet who visited earth and was unfamiliar with earth customs. The intrinsic information associated with an object can theoretically be figured out by examining the object itself.

A circle, though, may also have multiple *extrinsic* meanings, involving its relationships with other elements of the environment. For instance, the circle may symbolize a doughnut, an engagement ring, an inner tube flotation device, a part of the Olympic or a certain beer's logo, etc. Such "meanings" are not intrinsic to "circle" in the obvious sense that the "set of all points equidistant from a single point" is. The intrinsic meaning (the set of all points in the case of the circle) emerges from the points along the circle in a way that would be obvious to the space alien who had no contact with Earth society. The *extrinsic meanings* would not. The variable "X" may extrinsically refer to an infinite set of numbers or to variables such as prices, distances, times, etc. The quantity "5," though, includes the intrinsic meanings of "0 + 5, 1 + 4, and 2 + 3."

Words are examples of things that have extrinsic meanings. In itself, a word, e.g., "dog," has no intrinsic meaning. It does have specific extrinsic meaning in relationship to an outside pictorial dictionary which provides the key to its meaning. If one considers both the word and the dictionary together as a whole, then there becomes a specific intrinsic meaning to the "dog/dictionary" combination.

One should distinguish information from data. The individual points on the circle are data. The "circle" is something that emerges when all the points are in place and constitutes the information conveyed by the data. No single data point on the circle contains the information (meaning) of "circle." The circle is a meaning that emerges as a consequence of the data points being in place. Someone who travels on a circular road eventually arrives back at the starting point. This cyclic nature of a circle is an *emergent* property, dependent on the data points as a whole and is not a quality of any individual portion of a circle.

Thus, the meaning of an object or event depends on what the object or event refers to, and the meaning may be intrinsic (referring to the set of objects or events that comprise it) or extrinsic (referring to objects or events apart from the object itself).

The establishment of meaning does not necessarily require the presence of a human observer. The circle does not need a human observer to have the *intrinsic* meaning of a path without end. Similarly, words do not need a human observer to have *extrinsic* meaning in reference to an outside pictorial dictionary.

A Jonah-Mind can have as its basis either intrinsic or extrinsic information, as follows:

As in the story of Jonah-in-the-whale, there could be *intrinsic* information in regions of the brain that are inaccessible to the individual, conscious experiences of which the person is unaware. The individual cannot report such experiences, just as the whale cannot report Jonah's thoughts. Although the individual does not report the conscious experience, the consciousness nonetheless exists, as a Jonah-mind.

A Jonah-mind may also be based on *extrinsic* information. For instance, an individual may have heard the Chinese word for "dog" while having no idea as to the meaning of the word. The word, though, does relate to an outside Chinese pictorial dictionary and have an extrinsic meaning. If one considers the person's brain and the outside dictionary as a whole, there is a consciousness of the meaning of the word, but it is in the form of a Jonah-mind, an extrinsic meaning, which the person cannot report.

Information, whether intrinsic or extrinsic, can be considered a Jonah-mind if it is not reportable by the individual. Thus, if one considers two people standing together, one does not telepathically experience the thoughts of the other. One person's mind is a Jonah-mind in relation to the other.

CHAPTER 8.   CUSTOMARY CONSCIOUSNESS IN PART REQUIRES REPORTABLE INTRINSIC MEANING

I suggest that the "meaning" in our customary consciousness is an *intrinsic meaning*. If it were extrinsic, e.g., as in the meaning of a foreign word, which the person has heard but does not understand, the meaning would not be reportable by the individual. Meaning that is not reportable is a Jonah-mind, whether it is intrinsic meaning confined to a hidden recess of the brain and inaccessible to the individual, or is an extrinsic meaning that requires an outside dictionary or other translator to make sense. Thus, a person may know the Chinese word for "dog" but not know what it refers to, even though there may be an outside Chinese pictorial dictionary that shows the picture of a dog next to the word. The person could not, on just hearing the word, know to point to, or draw a dog to indicate that he knows the meaning. The Chinese word then has an extrinsic meaning of "dog," but not an intrinsic one.

The proposal in this book, then, is that customary human consciousness is information (meaning) in the brain, specifically the reportable intrinsic meaning associated with brain activity. The following thought experiment further examines the idea that any meaning of customary consciousness is intrinsic rather than extrinsic.

Elementary Computer Consciousness–a Paradox

Picture a very simple schematic of neuronal circuits in the brain that is set up to receive either light or sound stimuli. Imagine that a light in **Fig. 8–1A** shines on the retina. This leads to the relaying of impulses along the optic nerve (indicated by the arrow) to the visual area of the brain (VB). The subject is then asked to press one of two buttons (either "light" or "sound"), which will give us an indication as to what the person has experienced. In **Fig. 8–1A,** where there has been no re-arrangement of the circuits, the person will push the "light" button. When we ask him to tell us what he actually experienced consciously, he will say "light." Similarly, if a sound is played, the subject will press the "sound" button and say that he heard a sound.

In **Fig. 8–1B,** we have diverted the optic nerve to the auditory area of the brain (AB). In practice, this is not feasible since central nervous system axons do not re-

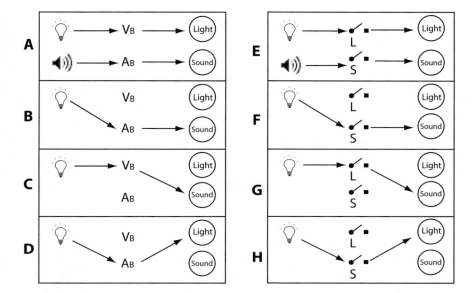

Figure 8-1

generate significantly, but let us imagine this hypothetically. Shining the light activates the auditory area of the brain. This will induce the person to push the "sound" button, just as he would if we were to stimulate the same area with electrodes. When we ask the person what he experienced, he will say, "sound," even though the original stimulus was the electromagnetic radiation that corresponds to light. We can readily understand this since the electromagnetic radiation of light is only a trigger that leads to the firing of the visual area of the brain, but here abnormally triggers the auditory area. One can accomplish the same effect by directly stimulating the auditory area of the brain with electrodes. The person will then report an auditory experience, regardless of whether or not (or how) the eyes connect with the brain.

In **Fig. 8–1C** we have twisted the person's peripheral nerves in a peculiar way so that a motor message originally intended to press the "light" button now ends up pressing the "sound" button. We now shine the light and observe the subject's response. The subject presses the "sound" button. We then ask the subject what he was conscious of, and he will say "I was conscious of the light and intended to press the light button, but strangely my hand ended up pressing the sound button by accident." We see a corresponding situation in real life in various clinical conditions: When peripheral nerves regenerate aberrantly, the resultant movement may not be that which was intended. In the phenomenon of *jaw-winking*, for instance, the subject intends to chew, but owing to aberrant growth of peripheral nerve fibers to the eyelid rather than the jaw muscles, he is forced to wink an eye in order to chew.

In **Fig. 8–1D** both the optic nerves and motor peripheral nerves have been crossed. When the light is shined, the person presses the "light" button but will report that he experienced sound and be perplexed as to why his hand pressed the wrong button.

In **Figs. 8–1A-D** we can see that the crucial events that relate to a person's verbal report of consciousness are occurring in the brain itself rather than in the peripheral levels of stimulus or response. If we totally eliminated the optic nerves and the peripheral "button-pressing" nerves and simply stimulated the visual area of the brain with an electrode, the person would have the conscious experience of light.

Now consider **Figs. 8–1E** through **H** in a very elementary computer that undergoes the same procedures. In this machine the mechanism in the "brain" is extraordinarily simple. It consists of a simple single switch. The light is shined on "light" receptors that convey electronic messages to the "light" area of the robot "brain" (L, the switch), resulting in the simple effect of flipping the single switch that leads to a robot arm pushing a "light" button. Since this is an extremely simple system, we do not have a complex speech function to tell us what "consciousness," if any, is actually experienced by the computer. We have to guess. Is there some sort of primitive consciousness associated with the light circuit that is different from consciousness associated with simulating the sound circuit? Now, no one would expect that there would be an experience of "light" or "sound" that resembled the experience of a person. But would there be any kind of consciousness, however simple, that differed between the L and S areas?

Let us first consider that there may be some difference in consciousness between the firing of the L ("light") and S ("sound") switches in the computer. What sort of consciousness would we expect in **Fig. 8–1F,** where the light and sound sensory paths are crossed? When light is presented in **Fig. 8–1F,** is the conscious experience of the L or the S variety? If the conscious experience occurs in the same manner as in series A-D, we would expect switch S to have an S type of consciousness and switch L to have an L type of consciousness when fired. Thus in **Fig. 8–1F,** where the light sensory pathway is crossed, we would expect an S type of consciousness on shining the light. In **Fig. 8–1G,** where the motor pathway is crossed, we would expect an L type of consciousness on shining the light. And in **Fig. 8–1H,** where both sensory and motor paths are crossed, we would expect an S type of consciousness on shining the light. But if so, examine **Figs. 8–1E** and **H** carefully. We are saying that the consciousness in response to light in **Fig. 8–1E** should be of the L type and the consciousness in **Fig. 8–1H** should be of the S type. But how can that be, when there is no fundamental difference between **Fig. 8–1E** and **H** except in terms of an irrelevant geometric twisting of the circuits? So one should *not* expect a difference in consciousness between L and H, while we do see a difference in the case of the brain. What accounts for this fundamental difference between brain and computer?

We can resolve this question by returning to the information content in the brain in **Figs. 8–1A** through **D.** There is a difference in information in V_B and A_B that is based on differences in wiring *within* the two brain areas, and this difference does not depend on the sensory or motor peripheral nerves. An electrode that stimulated a brain that was isolated in a vat would be expected to give rise to visual or auditory conscious experiences, depending on which brain region was picked. However, in **Figs. 8–1E-H,** there is no intrinsic difference between switches L and S. Stimulating them alone, out of context of the sensory or motor output, should give rise to no differences in consciousness.

When looked at as a *whole,* though, the entire light path, including the electromagnetic "light" waves, area L and the light button, does differ intrinsically from the entire sound path. However, the L and S regions have no intrinsic information that would distinguish the L region from the S region. In other words, if we just looked at a single switch firing, there would be no *intrinsic* difference in meaning between the activities of switches L and S. However, there is a difference in *extrinsic* meaning, in that the particular switch is part of the overall context of either the light or sound input.

Although the net result of just stimulating one switch or another would be the report of either "sound" or "light," this is just a report. There is no intrinsic difference between one switch and another. If the L and S regions were isolated from the environment and individually stimulated directly, there would be nothing about their firing that would suggest that there had to be some relationship between that firing and light or sound. Isolated firing of the L and S regions has no intrinsic meaning for light or sound.

Reportability is one ingredient necessary for customary consciousness, and there are reports of "sound" or "light" here in the case of the computer. However, there also has to be an intrinsic meaning in the mechanism that generates the report for there to be customary consciousness. Otherwise, any consciousness would be that of a Jonah-mind, rather than customary consciousness.

Looking at this from another perspective, imagine a situation where a computer was programmed to respond to many different kinds of inputs by merely storing in its memory a different number for the particular input, in no particular order. Thus, an input of the picture of a bird might generate the number 24387, a car 4937, a sound wave 58221, etc. The computer would be trained to respond with the words "bird," "car," "sound," etc., whenever the particular input was received or whenever one otherwise simply activated the areas of its circuits that stored the particular numbers. Would the computer actually be conscious (in the customary sense) of the bird, car, or sound? It would not, because although the reportability of the particular object is there, there is no intrinsic meaning to the numbers in themselves.

Customary consciousness, then, requires both reportability and intrinsic meaning.

Reportability without intrinsic meaning would not result in customary consciousness, although there may be a significant degree of Jonah-mind consciousness if one views the report in the context of an overall outside translating system that is unknown to the person. An example would be a person's memorizing a speech in a foreign language that he doesn't understand. There is significant extrinsic meaning to the word representations in his brain, but little intrinsic meaning, since they are only words.

Intrinsic meaning without reportability (e.g., in the so-called "unconscious" mind) would also not result in customary consciousness, although the degree of Jonah-mind consciousness may be significant. For instance, the person may undergo significant "unconscious" (actually Jonah-mind) thought processing without being able to report this. For a significant degree of customary consciousness, one needs both—reportability and intrinsic meaning.

Picture a paralyzed patient who cannot communicate with the outside world. Would that mean that he exhibits only a Jonah-mind while paralyzed, since he cannot issue a report? When the patient recovers and tells us that he was conscious all along, does that mean that it was not a Jonah-mind but his customary consciousness that he experienced while paralyzed? It makes no difference whether or not one calls his consciousness while paralyzed that of a Jonah-mind or that of customary consciousness. Both the Jonah-mind and customary consciousness are just as conscious. Relative to one person's mind, another person's mind is a Jonah-mind. What you call it depends on the context. The quality of the consciousness is the same, whether you call it Jonah-mind-type consciousness or our customary reportable consciousness.

There is one more requirement for customary consciousness, other than intrinsic meaning and reportability. Consider the situation where there is intrinsic meaning within the brain of person A, but the consciousness arises in a remote area of the brain that is not accessible for reporting. This would be a Jonah-mind form of consciousness since it is not reportable. But what if person B has a device that forces person A's vocal muscles to make the report, as if she were having an involuntary epileptic seizure. Person A would not feel she had the customary conscious experience, yet would be exhibiting reportability in the face of intrinsic meaning. There needs to be one more ingredient for customary consciousness, to be elaborated on in Chapter 11, in connection with the concept of "self."

CHAPTER 9.   HOW THE FIRING OF BRAIN CIRCUITS CAN HAVE INTRINSIC MEANING

One can understand how a circle can have the intrinsic meaning of the set of all points equidistant from a central point on a two-dimensional plane. One has only to examine the circle to determine this. But how can the firing of brain circuits, particularly in a hypothetical brain separated from its environment, have the intrinsic meaning of a particular sensation, thought process, feeling, or emotion? How could it do this without a translator?

In the field of code-breaking, the presumption is that for every code there is a hidden key necessary to interpret what the code refers to (Singh, '99). Sometimes one can figure out the key based on details within the code itself. For instance, in a coded paragraph consisting of substitute letters, the decoder may consider that in English (if it is an English language code) the most common letter is "e." The decoder may then assume that the most common letter referred to in the coded paragraph is "e." There are many other ways to try to find letter/word correlations in the coded message that correspond to those in the English language, and a code can often be broken without having the key in advance. But one still has to speculate on what the key might be and see if, on plugging it into the coded message, one gets a meaningful translation.

If the information in the human brain is in coded format, what is the key to its translation, and who is the translator? If the brain were simply a duplicating machine that precisely duplicated the outside environment, then one would not need a key to interpret any code, because there would be no code to interpret. However, the human brain does not appear to simply duplicate the outside environment. There is no picture projected onto a screen in the brain. The pattern of nerve impulses in the brain does not appear to resemble the outside environment. There would seem to be information in some sort of coded format, but what provides the interpretation of this code?

I suggest that the brain actually does duplicate the outside environment, not by projecting a movie picture, but by duplicating the associational relationships of the outside world, as follows:

We are used to thinking of the outside world as consisting of "things," such as houses, cars, rocks, etc. Let us shift our thinking to consider that rather than things, the outside world consists of *relationships*. Thus, consider a house. A house consists of doors, windows, walls, roof, etc. Each of these in turn consist of subdivisions of wood, glass, etc in particular geometric shapes. Ultimately all of these subdivisions reduce to molecules, atoms, and subatomic particles. In addition, all of the above have relationships with one another: the doors and windows in relationship to the walls, the walls in relationship to the roof and floor. The number of relationships among all of these is staggering, especially if one wants to consider the plumbing, electric wiring, appliances, etc., that go into the construction of a house. Now compare this to a cake. A particular cake may have a round shape, taste sweet, be soft, have layers of icing, perhaps chocolate, and texture, all of which differ from the hard wood and concrete of a house. One could draw a schematic of the myriad relationships for each.

The schematic drawing of relationships for "house" would not match that for "cake," even if couched in purely mathematical symbolic relationships. Even if we just drew lines to interconnect the relationships, without specifically mentioning the pictures or the words "icing" or "window", etc., the pattern of interrelationships in itself would differ significantly for "house" and "cake." Now just the word "house" or "cake" in itself, without any corresponding dictionary, would have no significant intrinsic meaning, and in itself would be ambiguous for any number of things (considering an infinite number of potential dictionaries). However, the more one considers not the words, but the associational relationships, the less ambiguous the meanings become. At a certain level of complexity, one could say that the meaning of the associations of "house" could not be interpreted as the meaning for "cake" or anything else.

Consider now the massive degree of complexity of the brain. We are dealing with some 10 to 100 billion neurons and some quadrillion synaptic connections in the brain. It has been estimated that if a different pattern of firing in the brain corresponded to a particular thought, then the number of possible thoughts that the human brain is capable of is somewhere near the number of atoms in the universe. (This sounds poetic, and may not be true, but the numbers are truly staggering!) The point is that the human brain is largely organized along unimaginably complex associational relationships (rather than just the storage of nonassociated data points).

The number and complexity of associations are so great that the meaning of a given pattern of firing, e.g. in the contemplation of "house," could not mean anything else but "house." If one were to imagine that the association meant "cake," the latter would necessitate an entirely different set of associations. The number and kind of associations needed to represent a cake would be entirely different from that needed to represent a house. The associations specific for house would differ from the associations for *anything* else, not just cakes. So there is within the brain an intrinsic meaning of "house" within the firing of the "house" circuits. A key and a translator are not necessary, such as a dictionary would be needed to translate a word. The meaning of the outside environment is duplicated by duplicating within the brain the relationships of the outside world.

This does not mean that there is a physical world of houses and cakes inside the brain, any more than it would mean that a holographic image of a house or cake contains an actual physical house or cake. The holographic image contains the concept of house or cake, but not the actual physical house or cake, since the underlying molecules that constitute house or cake are not present. Similarly, in the brain, the duplicated associations do not cause a duplicated physical environment, but do represent the concept of the house or cake.

One may object to the suggestion that the essence of reality consists of relationships rather than the "objects" themselves. That is, there do appear to be real objects in the outside world that happen to have relationships, and that, without the objects, the brain does not really have the representation of the outside environment. However, when we consider what "objects" are, such as houses and cars, they themselves can be considered to consist of relationships among objects. The car consists of motor, wheels, steering wheel, etc. But each of these car parts also consist of relationships, all the way down to the atomic level. When we consider this vast array of relationships, and consider that in the end they reduce to relationships of atoms in space and time, we have to ask whether or not we really need the actual atoms in order to arrive at the concept of car. A holograph or ordinary film can capture the concept of car without having to include the atoms, but only needs the higher levels of the hierarchical relationships. The brain, by duplicating the upper level of the hierarchy of environmental relationships, thus provides meaning, which is consciousness.

I should like to be clear about the use of the term "environment." By that, I mean not just the world outside the body, but all the parts of the body that connect with the brain, bringing to the brain data about the body itself, such as a geometric map of the body surface and the workings of the internal organs. The intrinsic information in the brain is derived partly from data received from the internal and external environment of the body, through learning since birth. The intrinsic information in the brain also arises in part through heredity, whereby relationships that promoted survival became affixed in the brain through evolution.

Not Functionalism

Consciousness in this book is viewed as intrinsic information, as intrinsic meaning. This idea of consciousness should not be viewed as falling into the philosophical classification that is termed "functionalism." "Functionalism" implies some sort of extrinsic functional relationship between the brain and its surrounding environment. Thus, in functionalism the meaning of what happens in the brain is the direct result of what those firing circuits accomplish in their final motor output. Or, the meaning refers to the meaning of the specific sensory input to the brain from the outside environment. This meaning would not exist in an isolated brain kept in a vat. Thus, the meaning of what is embedded on a music CD is based on the premise that the CD will ultimately connect with speakers that will cause air wave vibrations that stimulate the eardrum and finally the brain. The meaning of what is on the CD also relates to the fact that the original recording came from musical instruments. Without knowledge of such recording input, and in the absence of any output to speakers, what is on the CD does not necessarily relate to music or sound. It could just as well have the meaning of patterns of light if the CD were connected to a light-patterning output device. Thus, the meaning of the CD relates to its function. Such is not true of the brain. A brain isolated in a vat, with no sensory or motor input, and incapable of demonstrating communication with the outside world, should still exhibit consciousness when stimulated, solely on the basis of the firing patterns of its neurons.

In a patient with quadriplegia from interruption of the connections between the brain and body below the head, the brain maintains the same ability to think and contemplate the areas of the body below the head. Patients who are blind or deaf can still contemplate visual images and music. Electrode stimulation of the brain will produce conscious experiences, and there is every reason to believe that such experiences would arise even if the brain were isolated from the environment. Thus, rather than representing functionalism, the theory of consciousness in this book is based on intrinsic information in the brain irrespective of the brain's functional relationships with the environment outside the brain. That intrinsic information is postulated to arise from associational relationships within the brain.

CHAPTER 10. CONSCIOUSNESS AND AMBIGUITY OF MEANING

As the complexity of associations increases in the brain, the meaning of those associations becomes less ambiguous. Conversely, if one reduces the complexity of a brain to a few connections, the ambiguity is high. Thus, the intrinsic meaning of a single isolated neuronal connection is small, but its extrinsic meaning is virtually infinite, just as the letter "X" can have an infinite number of extrinsic meanings. While there can be a vast number of circuit firing patterns whose meanings are unambiguous, there may be others for which there is some measure of ambiguity. What would consciousness be like in that case? Would the person be aware of both meanings or neither?

Consider, for instance, that sound "hee," which means "he" in English, but "she" in Hebrew. If the person is of English background and has the details of the English dictionary translation in his brain, then in *association* with that internal dictionary, the "hee"/dictionary association carries the intrinsic meaning of male. Similarly, if the person carries in mind the details of a Hebrew dictionary, then the "hee"/Hebrew dictionary association carries the intrinsic meaning of female. If there is neither dictionary in mind, and the person doesn't know either English or Hebrew, then the meaning of "hee" is ambiguous, and there is no customary consciousness of either gender. However, even if "hee" alone is ambiguous, the sound still has extrinsic meaning of male in respect to an English dictionary in the outside environment and the extrinsic meaning of female in respect to a Hebrew dictionary in the outside environment, and an infinite number of other extrinsic meaning in relationship to an infinite number of other potential dictionaries. These extrinsic meanings constitute Jonah-mind consciousness. In itself, though, "hee" does not have such meaning intrinsically, and the person would not define the word as referring to either male or female, or both, or anything else, without being exposed to the dictionary definition.

Thus, if consciousness is meaning, and the person does not know English or Hebrew, there is still a form of consciousness of both male and female in respect to the sound "hee," but that consciousness is in the form of a Jonah-mind, being hidden, in this case based on extrinsic meanings. For customary consciousness to exist, there needs to be intrinsic meaning within the brain, along with reportability.

CHAPTER 11. INTRINSIC MEANING, REPORTABILITY, AND "SELF CIRCUITS" AS THE KEY REQUIREMENTS FOR CUSTOMARY CONSCIOUSNESS

In addition to intrinsic meaning and reportability, there is a further factor needed for customary consciousness. As a thought experiment, consider a brain that has within it the intrinsic meaning of "tree," but this information resides in an isolated area of the brain that does not communicate with anything outside itself. The person does not report the thought of "tree," even though the circuits for this are firing in the isolated area. We would say that there is intrinsic consciousness of tree, but it is of the Jonah-mind variety, because it is not reportable.

What if, though, an outside source manipulated the person's nervous system, like a puppet, and forced the vocal cords to respond "tree" to the question of what the person was thinking. Then there would be the intrinsic meaning of "tree" in the brain as well as the vocal report to the outside world of "tree." Would this constitute customary consciousness? It would not, because the reportability needs to be coming from the "person" himself to be categorized as the human variety of customary consciousness. Otherwise, the person would say that he was forced, like a puppet, to utter the word "tree" but wasn't thinking about a tree. But who is "the person"?

With virtually every interaction that a person has throughout life with the body's inside and outside environment, that information relates in some way to the information about the body itself. All this information about the body becomes consolidated into one category of meaning that may be termed the "self." For a person to be customarily conscious of "tree," the "tree" circuitry would need to be associated with the "self" circuitry in such a manner that the "self"/"tree" circuits can report on the presence of "tree" information. The *report* would need to convey the (*intrinsic*) information that "I" have recognized the "tree" for there to be customary consciousness. The report needs to be made by the "self" circuits so that the person can say "I saw that." Performing the trick of manipulating the vocal cords to report this, like a puppet, does not satisfy this requirement. To do so only shows that one can fool other people into thinking the person (or advanced robot) is conscious of "tree" when actually he is not. The person himself will express surprise that his vocal cords suddenly expressed the word "tree." To the person, that report is more like an epileptic seizure or the involuntary outcry of a person with Tourette's syndrome.

Thus, customary consciousness requires intrinsic meaning, reportability, and the added ingredient of the "self" circuitry of the brain.

CHAPTER 12.   THE HIERARCHICAL
STRUCTURE OF MEANING

But what is it that creates the conscious experience of "red" or "sweet" or "smell of coffee," or the emotions of fear, love, happiness and sadness? Part of the difficulty in understanding how these qualia can originate from the firing of neuronal circuits is our impression that sensations such as color, sound, smell, taste, or pain are singular entities that cannot be subdivided further. We only sense the overall qualia rather than what may be subdivisions of the qualia.

As physics and chemistry have evolved, scientists have found that many of the elements of nature can be reduced to simpler ones. Myriad kinds of molecules can be reduced to a relatively small number of kinds of atoms, which can be reduced to more basic ingredients, such as electrons, protons, and neutrons. These subatomic entities are similar in all molecules but create much molecular diversity in the right combinations. Combining the basic elements in different ways leads to the emergence of different molecules with diverse properties, even though the underlying structural ingredients are the same.

Physicists now see the forces of nature as simpler and less diverse than previously thought. Rather than postulating totally separate forces for wind, rain, fire, lightning, etc., physics has moved toward a unification of relatively few primary forces of nature. Electricity and magnetism have fused into a single entity of electromagnetism. Energy and mass are interconvertible. Some physicists suggest that mass may be a distortion of space. The forces of gravity, magnetism, and the strong and weak forces of the atomic world are considered to be spinoffs of a more primary force. Time and space have become fused into a singular spacetime.

With the progressive simplification of the forces of nature into a few primary entities, it would be strange to find that conscious experiences such as "red," "C sharp," "sweet," "smell of rose," and pain (and whatever other kinds of conscious experiences exist throughout the animal kingdom) are each primary entities with no further subdivisions. It is natural to wonder whether these conscious experiences are themselves subdividable into more primary conscious entities, which when combined can lead to the emergence of new kinds of meanings, in the form of vision, hearing, taste, smell, and touch. A house emerges from the juxtaposition of its walls, ceilings, windows, and doors. These consist of molecules, which in turn consist of atoms, which consist of primary particles. We can appreciate the house arising from primary particles when we see all the intermediate levels from primary particle to house. It would be difficult to appreciate how a house related to primary particles if one could not see the intermediate levels but could only see the quantum mechanics of subatomic particles. We may have a similar difficulty in trying to understand the origin of human sensory experiences. We experience the final emergent product (the "red," the "taste," like we do the "house") but cannot experience the underlying subdivisions of "red" or "taste." Those may be Jonah-minds. Only the final emergent product, the "red," is experienced in customary consciousness, which can make the report. Simpler subdivisions of consciousness might not be experienced in our customary consciousness, since they may be Jonah-minds.

Does this mean that there is some primary irreducible root, or "quark" of consciousness, from which all the conscious experiences are built, like a Lego set? One would still have to explain what gave that elementary unit the quality of consciousness in the first place, however elementary it might be.

Perhaps a better way of looking at this is to consider an elementary relationship, for instance the connection between one neuron and another. In a sense, the meaning of such a simple connection is highly ambiguous, much as the letter "X" has infinite ambiguity as to what "X" stands for, whether some number or parameter such as space, time, apples, or dollars. The elementary relationship between two neurons has little intrinsic meaning, but a great deal of extrinsic meaning, much as the simple letter "X" could stand for anything. Meanings become less ambiguous (acquire more intrinsic meaning) as more connections are added, until a point is reached in which the myriad interconnections can only refer in their intrinsic meaning to something highly specific and complex, whether it is a static image or sequence of events. Thus, while consciousness always exists at every level of complexity, it proceeds from lower levels that are highly ambiguous (extrinsic meanings), representing essentially extrinsic information, to levels that are highly specific, representing significant intrinsic information. That intrinsic information gains the quality of customary consciousness when it becomes reportable by the individual.

As a more specific example of a low level of meaning, consider the equation $y = mx + b$, which is the equation for a straight line. Intrinsically, it does not contain the *visual* information of a straight line, but it does portray *linearity*. The equation $y = mx2 + b$ (the formula for a parabola) does not portray the visual information for a parabola, but does convey information about a certain nonlinearity. A fractal equation (e.g., $z = x + ji$, where i refers to an imaginary number, the square root of minus 1) contains a vast amount of detailed information when laid out as a two-dimensional fractal graphic. It does not in itself portray the visual image of a fractal picture, but it does have great meaning in itself, if only in the geometric mathematical format.

I propose that there is such an elementary "quark" of consciousness, a building block for higher levels, but, rather than a subatomic particle, it is in the form of a very low level of meaning. We have difficulty conceiving what such a low level of meaning must be like, since trying to think about it inevitably leads one to use much higher levels of meaning in the consideration, such as the concept of one's "self." High levels of meaning (color, sound, etc.) emerge from lower levels of meaning that do not resemble the higher levels any more than a point on a circle resembles the circle.

If one tries to dissect the overall customary conscious experience into simple subcomponents, one may find subcomponents which in themselves are highly specific representations of environmental relationships and have their own intrinsic meanings. Those subcomponents, however, do not carry the meaning of the whole, just as an arc within the circumference of a circle does not carry the meaning of an unending path. Further subdivisions result in less and less complex meaning and more ambiguity until the definitive intrinsic meaning is so minimal as to be intrinsically almost "meaningless."

I offer the following speculative examples to give an idea as to how the higher levels of meaning might emerge from lower levels.

Regarding pain, consider a simple reaction to a noxious stimulus, an amoeba withdrawing its pseudopod in response to a micro pinprick. There is no suggestion that the amoeba is thinking: "That hurt. I'd better withdraw this part of my body." Yet something is happening, a biochemical reaction, which through evolution has led (perhaps for survival value) to the withdrawal of the pseudopod. Perhaps the withdrawal in this situation is a type of *protopain,* not resembling true pain, but one of the simplest elements of it, a survival activity in response to a potentially harmful stimulus. Combine this primitive protopain with higher elements, in vertebrates for instance, which fuse this meaning with the idea of localization to a particular area of the body map, and the meaning becomes more complex. Perhaps there are many other elements as well, neural circuits and chemicals to induce a reaction to run away ("flight or fight" response), to change blood pressure and pulse, etc. A whole host of body reactions combine to form the meaning of it all put together. There then emerges the experience of "localized pain," which is difficult for the individual to dissect much further, since the subdivisions are Jonah-minds.

Regarding color, the wavelength of red is not "red" (the wavelength could just as well generate heat, when delivered via a laser). It is a trigger to the nervous system. When we see "red," the meanings that arise in the nervous system include such submeanings as "associated with the eyes," "disappears on closing the eyes," "not something that can be touched directly even though associated with objects," "not associated with the ears or other sense organs," etc. But why specifically "red" and not another color? If we could individually experience all of the submeanings that construct the "red" experience, we might get a better idea as to why the experience had to be a "red" one. Or perhaps we could never understand, since the submeanings would remain hidden as Jonah-minds. Or we might not be able to comprehend such submeanings because the experience of "red," being the emergent property of simpler submeanings, might disappear when we try to dissect the experience into simpler components. The simpler components would not in themselves have the emergent property of "red," just as an individual point on a circle does not carry the meaning of an "unending path."

Primary components of the atomic structure can give rise to the higher order emergent principles and rules of cell biology, physiology, anatomy, and psychology (**Fig. 12–1**), which are difficult to comprehend in terms of the primary elements alone. Similarly, it may not be possible to jump from understanding the lower primary submeanings of consciousness at the cellular level directly up to the higher emergent level of "red." Trying to understand consciousness by contemplating neuronal connection activity may be like trying to contemplate a house by contemplating the quantum mechanical associations of primary particles in the brick molecules. The lowest level of neuronal activity may have an elementary level of intrinsic meaning (and vast extrinsic meaning) associated with it, but that intrinsic meaning would not resemble the higher level consciousness of vision, sound, taste, smell, touch, or other customary conscious experience.

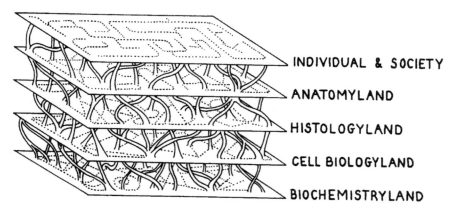

INDIVIDUAL & SOCIETY

ANATOMYLAND

HISTOLOGYLAND

CELL BIOLOGYLAND

BIOCHEMISTRYLAND

Figure 12-1

CHAPTER 13.   THE INTRINSIC
ORIGIN OF THE SENSES

It is relatively easy for us to consider taste and smell as originating in the nervous system and not in the molecules that act as triggers to the nervous system. After all, why should a simple molecule intrinsically carry the information of "taste of coffee" or "smell of rose "? One can understand that such conscious experiences arise from activity within the nervous system rather than from the molecular triggers of taste and smell that activate the taste and smell receptors in the tongue and nose. Electrode stimulation of the appropriate brain area could elicit the same conscious experience. It is also easy to see how "touch" or "pain" are not intrinsic to the feather or pin that trigger the nervous system's touch and pain receptors, but are experiences that arise from within.

One can even, with a little more consideration, understand that sound does not exist outside the body within what are just vibrating air waves. The "sound" waves are just triggers to the nervous system, where the experience of sound is created. The sound waves may carry spatiotemporal information that characterizes, say, a particular piece of music, but it requires the brain to make sound and music out of that pattern. (Thus, when no one is around, a sound is not made when a tree falls in the forest!) The same air waves could just as well trigger pain in the ears if intense enough. These sensations would also not exist alone in the forest.

What needs a bit more pondering to appreciate is the idea that vision similarly does not arise in the outside environment. We believe that what we see in the outside environment really exists visually. If it didn't exist, we would wonder whether there were any reality at all outside us, since so much of our consciousness presents itself in visual terms. However, the experience of vision may be no different from that of sound, taste, smell, or touch, in that it may arise solely within the brain. This does not mean that light waves act solely as triggers to the nervous system. On striking the retina, light waves also carry spatiotemporal information, but not necessarily that of vision—more of a geometrical mathematical nature. That is, a person who can only experience touch, but is blind since birth, may recognize the geometry of his outside environment through touch and not be able to conceive of things in visual terms. Space in the outside environment need not be intrinsically visual any more than it is intrinsically tactile. Perhaps the geometry exists in the outside world, and light waves carrying that information trigger the nervous system, but do not contain the information in visual format. It is up to the brain, through association with the body map and concept of "eyes," to add the conscious experience of "sight" to the geometric spatiotemporal information that does enter the nervous system.

The environment, then, provides meaning in terms of time and space, conveying information about space in neither visual, aural, tactile, or other format, but rather in a mathematical format. The brain provides the meaning of sight, sound, taste, smell, and touch. The meanings of the latter senses do not arise within the triggers to the nervous system (the incoming light waves, sound waves, molecules of rose in the air, molecules of coffee on the tongue, or the pin or feather). The meanings of the senses arose partly through learning and partly through evolution, which through the millennia resulted in the adaptation of the organism to its environment. Evolution provided the organism with the qualities of life (organization, movement, irritability, growth, adaptation, reproduction), a body map and the means therewith to distinguish self from outside environment. The construction of the nervous system and its manner of functioning has great meaning within itself at birth. The environment after birth provides additional meaning in terms of spatial and temporal mathematical relations of the environment, and also provides triggers to the already ingrained information within the nervous system.

In summary, the sensory experiences of sight, vision, smell, taste, and touch arise within the nervous system rather than in the outside world. These senses are not singular irreducible entities. Each is the emergent property of many subdivisions, which in themselves are Jonah-minds, not reportable and not part of customary consciousness. The further one dissects the conscious experience into its subcomponents, the more ambiguous the meanings of the subcomponents become. As subcomponents of meaning combine, there emerges a more complex structure of overall meaning that is less ambiguous (more intrinsic in meaning) than its subcomponents. The circuitry patterns that are associated with the individual senses arose partly through evolution and partly through learning after birth. The intrinsic meaning that we are looking for in the activity of the brain can be found in the complex patterns of interactions of the brain, which intrinsically refer to specific images and event associations in the environment, whether acquired through learning or heredity.

CHAPTER 14.   EXPLAINING CLASSIC PROBLEMS IN THE FIELD OF CONSCIOUSNESS

With the preceding discussion, a number of classic issues in the field of consciousness become more readily understandable.

The Binding Problem

Describing consciousness as "meaning" can resolve the "binding problem." Considerable activity occurs in a brain in both space and time during the execution of a thought. Contemplating the picture of a tiger, for instance, involves neuronal firing on a large scale in both space and time. The "binding problem" is the dilemma as to why so many isolated neuronal firings in the brain, not only separated in space, but also in time, should appear to be bound into a single conscious experience. We see the "tiger" as a whole rather than many isolated bits of information.

The holistic nature of quantum mechanics has been suggested as a way to resolve the binding problem. For instance, in quantum mechanics two particles may be identical except for their having an opposite "spin." When separated by far distances, the two particles may show a kind of binding together (also called *entanglement*). When the direction of spin of one particle is determined, the direction of spin of the other particle becomes immediately determined, even if the latter particle is light-years away. According to quantum physicists the direction of spin of the particles is not just unknown prior to the observation. There *is* no direction until the observation is made. Thus, there is a binding that can exist across great distances.

Some scientists have suggested that quantum interactions at the submicroscopic neuronal cell level (e.g., microtubules) account for the binding of consciousness (Penrose, '94). This hypothesis, though, seems very much at the wrong level of organization. It is like proposing that quantum interactions in the structure of metal are responsible for the concept of a car. The concept of a car depends on the associations at a much higher level of macrostructures, such as engines, batteries, pipes, wheels, and wires, and their interconnections. Similarly, consciousness, if it is contingent on the pattern of associations among neurons, likely depends on the much more macroscopic interactions of neural networks and their meaning, irrespective of the underlying mechanisms of individual cell biochemistry and biophysics. Biochemistry and biophysics serve the more microscopic functions of preserving individual cell integrity, producing and transporting neurotransmitter molecules, and relaying individual electrochemical communications at the cellular level. If consciousness depends on the patterns of interneuronal connections, it should exist even if the carriers of the information are not biological.

There is a fallacy to the view that the holistic quality of quantum mechanics is necessary to explain the binding of consciousness. Some scholars claim that classical physics cannot explain binding, i.e., that classical physics can only describe a collection of objects as isolated unbound entities, whereas quantum mechanics can bind them (Stapp, '93). This is not so, for a collection of objects can have *meaning* irrespective of quantum mechanics. Meaning alone is a type of binding, and if consciousness is meaning, then *there is no need to postulate anything other than meaning alone to account for the binding of consciousness.* The events in the brain involving neuronal firing over different distances and different times can have an overall meaning. *Meaning alone can suffice for the binding of consciousness.*

The Chinese Room Issue

The *Chinese Room* issue (Searle, '92) is an argument that has been used to dispute the idea that computers can be conscious. In this thought experiment, a subject who does not understand Chinese is given questions in Chinese to answer in Chinese. Although the subject does not understand Chinese, he somehow (hypothetically, of course) has memorized the correct answers in Chinese, or has someone who knows Chinese (or a detailed phrase book) tell him all the correct answers in Chinese to any question that might be asked of him in Chinese. He answers correctly, but without understanding the meaning of what he is saying. To an outside observer, the subject seems to be completely fluent in Chinese and appears to understand what he is saying. The observer comes to the false conclusion that the subject knows the meaning of his words, even though the subject hasn't the foggiest idea of what they mean. He might say the Chinese word for "dog," but have no idea that it refers to "dog," be unable to point to a dog, or draw a picture of a dog, to indicate that he knows the meaning of the Chinese word. This thought experiment has been used to suggest two points about computers and consciousness:

1. Although a computer might appear to simulate human thought, this does not mean that the computer is conscious, in the customary sense, of the meaning of what it is conveying.
2. Computers cannot be conscious, because all a computer deals with are symbols (*syntax*). And symbols, such as words, do not in themselves convey their meaning (*semantics*). It requires a human interpreter to achieve meaning and consciousness of that meaning. In philosophical jargon, "Syntax is not sufficient for semantics."

The preceding discussions are consistent with conclusion 1. Just saying words does not mean that the speaker, or the computer, experiences the meaning of what he/it is saying. Words are only triggers and do not have intrinsic meaning. However, conclusion 2, that a computer cannot be conscious, is mistaken. It sets up the straw man, portraying the computer as only capable of processing and giving its output in the form of words and symbols. We know that words are only triggers. Words do not intrinsically contain the real information behind them. We would not expect a computer that dealt with just spitting out words by rote in response to questions to be conscious (in the customary sense) of much.

There is a big difference between recording information as words and recording it as complex circuitry interrelationships that relate to, and duplicate, associative relationships of the environment. A computer could, in principle, have those complex associations. Like the computer, our own brains contain information in the form of symbols, but the interrelationships of those symbols provide intrinsic meaning. Those associative connections in the brain are far more meaningful (intrinsically) than just words. It is not the fact that present-day computers deal with mathematical symbols that prevent them from having significant consciousness. The information in our own brains is also represented by symbols of a mathematical nature in the form of the pluses and minuses of synaptic stimulation and inhibition. What is important is whether the interconnections among those mathematical symbols duplicate the relationships of the outside environment. It is the meaning of those relationships that constitutes consciousness. A computer can be conscious if it has the right interrelationships within its circuitry. Even present-day computers are conscious to the simple degree that their complex associations suggest.

If the person in the Chinese room experiment correctly stated, in response to the Chinese word for "dog," another Chinese word that was synonymous for dog, the same person would still not be able to point to a real dog, or draw a dog, to indicate that he understood what was being said. However, if the person could also respond by drawing *a picture* of a dog at the same time, this would give more indication that he was really conscious of the meaning of the word. The mistake that has been made in interpreting the Chinese room experiment is the assumption that a computer cannot be conscious because it only deals with symbols. But if the relationships and interactions among the symbols are sufficiently sophisticated that they intrinsically represent only certain events in the environment, there can be customary consciousness.

Even if words are the only form of communication in the Chinese room experiment, there would still be an extrinsic consciousness of the meaning of the words, since the words refer to a hidden potential pictorial dictionary. One should not be so hasty to dismiss the idea of "the room" being consciousness. Perhaps a better way of putting it: There is an extrinsic consciousness, actually an infinite number of extrinsic consciousnesses, for each of the words, depending on which potential dictionary is used, regardless of how far the dictionary is from the person uttering the word. The person would not be aware of the meaning of the word (in the customary sense of consciousness), but such consciousness would nonetheless exist in extrinsic form.

Thus, we might be fooled into thinking that a cleverly designed talking computer had customary consciousness of what it is saying, but the fact that it responds correctly to questions, like a human being, does not mean that it really has such customary consciousness. Outputting words alone is insufficient for a computer to be conscious in the customary sense. However, computers may eventually reach a high level of consciousness, conceivably even more than that of humans, by duplicating the associations of the outside environment.

Split-Brain Experiments

Neurosurgeons, in rare cases of epilepsy, have tried to sever all lines of communication between the right and left hemispheres of the brain (Gazzaniga et al, '62) to prevent epileptic attacks from spreading from one hemisphere to the other. Superficially, the patients later appeared normal. However, more detailed studies on such patients produced striking evidence of independent functioning of the hemispheres.

In most people, the left cerebral hemisphere controls speech function, and each hemisphere controls motor activity on the opposite side of the body. A split-brain patient, when presented, through elaborate testing devices, with a picture of a spoon to the left visual field (which connects to the nondominant right cerebral hemisphere) actually might say (using his dominant left hemisphere) that he was unaware of any picture. At the same time the right hemisphere would direct the patient's left hand to point out the spoon and clearly indicate its awareness of the spoon. Each half of the brain is rendering a different opinion of what lies before it.

This situation is easily understood through the Jonah-mind principle. Both hemispheres contribute to consciousness. The surgical splitting of the brain into two independently functioning hemispheres, each of which communicates separately with the outside world, results in the appearance to the observer of two separate conscious entities. This should not be surprising, since we normally have many conscious Jonahs inside of us according to the Jonah-mind principle. The body cannot report to the outside world about the consciousness of its Jonahs, but normally acts as a single functioning unit to tell the outside world about its customary consciousness. It therefore typically appears to an observer that there is only one conscious mind. It should not be surprising that we find in the split-brain experiments two conscious entities, each unaware of the other, associated with the same individual. The appearance of two conscious entities occurs because the two hemispheres independently communicate with the outside world, rather than with themselves, presenting themselves as two functioning units, rather than one. Each hemisphere may be customarily conscious but is a Jonah-mind to the other hemisphere, just as Jonah is unable to communicate with the whale, and just as one person is unaware of another's consciousness.

If one semantically defines "consciousness as" requiring speech (as some people do), then one would consider only the dominant hemisphere as conscious in the split-brain studies. However, if one regards consciousness as "meaning" (information), and admits that meaning (information) can be communicated to the outside world not only through speech but also through body language, then since both hemispheres communicate to the outside world they are not only conscious, but conscious in the customary sense. Our customary consciousness is likely far more developed than that of other animals simply because we do have a better means of communicating it, through speech.

Blindsight

The Jonah-mind principle provides a ready understanding of the phenomenon of *blindsight*. Patients with this disorder believe they are blind, but can correctly identify an object that is shown to them, suggesting they detect the visual stimuli that are presented to them (Dennett, '91; Baars, '97). It is as if they are unconscious of the visual presentation, yet act as if they do know about them. The Jonah-mind principle regards blindsight simply as a situation where visual data are processed in a Jonah-mind. The results of that processing are then relayed to the customary conscious mind, which gives the report.

The Idiot Savant

An *idiot savant,* while showing severe mental dysfunction, may have extraordinary talents in certain very specific areas. For instance, the savant may be able to multiply in his mind a fifty-digit number by another fifty-digit number and come up with the correct answer. The fascinating feature is that the person may not be able to tell you how he did it. The Jonah-mind principle would regard this as an instance of mathematical calculation occurring within a Jonah-mind, which in turn gives the results to the customary conscious mind, a situation similar to that of blindsight. Much of what we call "intuition" or the "ah-hah!" revelation may operate on a similar principle; there is much Jonah-mind information processing, with only the end result coming to customary consciousness.

Mary, the Colorblind Physiologist

The hypothetical case of Mary, the colorblind physiologist (Jackson, '86), has been used to suggest that consciousness must involve more than the functional processing of the brain, but this reasoning is flawed. The argument asks one to consider Mary, a world-class neurophysiologist who know everything there is to know about the brain and its functioning, including all the neural processing that goes on while one contemplates a color. The only problem is that Mary is colorblind since birth. Can she teach herself to see color by contemplating all the functioning of the brain that goes on during the conscious experience of seeing color? No, she cannot, so the argument goes that there must be more to seeing color than just the firing of circuits in the brain. This reasoning is flawed, however, for a number of reasons:

- Consciousness of color is not the same as the carrier of color information (the brain). It is the information itself that resides in the brain. Trying to contemplate that information by thinking about the anatomy of neuronal circuits mistakes the carrier of the information (the brain itself) for the information itself.

- The only way for Mary to experience the color is for the circuits in her nervous system to fire in a similar way as those of a person who can see color, having both the same intrinsic meaning as well as reportability. But Mary's nervous system is defective in that way. The photoreceptors of Mary's retina do not function in a way that can relay the proper sequence of nerve impulses from the retina to the brain. Nor are the relationships within the brain circuits in the visual areas of her brain set up to be able to interpret such information or to fire that way, even when stimulated through electrodes. Showing Mary what the pattern of neuronal impulses looks like in the brain of a person with color vision, does not fire the same circuits that must fire in order to see color (the same arguments as for **Fig. 3–2**). So she cannot see color regardless of how much she learns about the functioning of the brain in a person who can see color.

- Color, as discussed above, is not a singular entity but a very complex conscious experience, structured from many lower levels of meaning. It would be impossible for Mary to picture in her mind all the complex neuronal connection associations that must come into play for the structuring of the meaning of a color. The human mind can only experience a small amount of customary consciousness at a given time. Picturing less than the full structure of the circuitry that gives rise to the color experience would not produce the experience of color any more than picturing a small part of a circle would give rise to an understanding of the "never-ending" path quality of a circle. The experience of color emerges from lower levels of organization that in themselves do not constitute color.

Reversed Qualia

It is an old question as to whether or not the qualia that other people experience are similar to one's own. For instance, does one person see "red" in the same way as another person? Is it even possible that the "red-orange-yellow-blue-indigo-violet" sequence seen by one person from top to bottom on a rainbow pattern in the sky could actually be seen in reverse sequence for another person? In such case, the latter person might experience the qualia in reverse: seeing violet at the top but calling it red, and seeing red at the bottom but calling it violet.

Certainly, we know that all people do not experience color the same way. The most obvious example is that of colorblindness, where some individuals have great difficulty in distinguishing red and green, or blue and yellow. And there are also more subtle examples besides that of colorblindness. As a personal example, I am not colorblind, but my sensitivity to green is less than that of my wife. Thus, in a dim light I see my raincoat as gray, whereas Harriet sees it as green, which I require better lighting in order to see. It is not only in the area of color vision that people differ. For instance, about one fourth of people in the United States cannot, on a hereditary basis, taste the bitter substance called phenylthiocarbamid (PTC).

Putting aside these clear differences in the way people see colors, is it possible that people really experience different colors even when they do not report differences in their experiences? In some respects we can confirm that some aspects of color vision are consistent from one person to another. We can show this when different individuals report on the *relationships* between the color experiences. For instance, two observers may agree that "orange" lies between "red" and "yellow." They may agree on the relationships. In that respect, the color experiences appear to be similar (Churchland, '02).

Beyond that, can we say anything further about whether or not different people have common experiences in describing a particular color or other conscious experience? From the point of view expressed in this book, it is the *relationships* that define the specific nature of the qualia. Hence, if the relationships are the same, the actual conscious experiences should be the same, and we can go a little further in suggesting that it is likely that people who report common relationships within the conscious experience have similar conscious experiences. However, we cannot say for sure that the experiences are identical, because many of the lower hierarchical "relationships" that constitute a color or other experience may be in the form of Jonah-minds, and are not describable. Without being able to report the nature of these lower hierarchical relationships, there remains the possibility that experiences of color between two individuals might still differ, despite their identical reports of other aspects of their color experiences.

Novel Qualia

Can a person experience a categorically different kind of sensation, other than that of sight, hearing, smell, taste, and touch (e.g., like echolocalization in the bat)? Since it is relationships that matter, altering the brain circuitry or electrical stimulation to form different relationships could, in principle, produce different categories of sensory experience. Moods and emotions are strange mixes of a great variety of information, so one may well experience a new type of mood or emotional experience. Strikingly new experiences can occur under the influence of hallucinogenic agents.

Consciousness of Self

A number of authors define consciousness as "awareness of self" and consider this the critical issue in understanding consciousness. In this book, consciousness is simply defined as awareness or, better, the experience of "red," "taste of coffee," etc., without necessitating having to think about "self" at the same time.

Consciousness of self is a complex form of consciousness specific to humans and perhaps certain other animals. Understanding how consciousness of self arises becomes much simpler after understanding how consciousness itself arises. The preceding chapters have presented an explanation for how consciousness arises, not requiring "self" for consciousness per se to exist. Consciousness is something that permeates nature. How does consciousness of "self" arise? The simplest explanation is that a critical part of the setup of the human nervous system is a map of the individual's body, the representation within the brain of the body's surface and internal anatomy. Throughout life, whenever any input reaches the brain, it is associated with this map – vision is associated with the eyes, smell with the nose, etc. The sense of self gradually develops as the child explores his/her body. Every sensation is related to the map of the whole body in the brain. So the experience of "red" becomes the experience of "red that I see." "I" is not some different mystic dimension outside the brain and body. It is similar to any other information in the brain, but in the case of "I," it is information about the body that is associated with the experiences. "Self" is then one more item of information that the brain stores, but it is the most frequently accessed item, the one with the most far-reaching associative connections in the brain. The "self" circuits are associated continually with the sensory input, information processing and motor output of the brain.

Consciousness of Consciousness

If consciousness is meaning, how does the brain know about this meaning so as to be able to say, "That is a red apple, and I am aware that I am aware of this"?

The brain consists of myriad individual nerve cells, each doing its robotic function, which Minsky ('85) has termed "agents." The collective activity of all those neurons produces the response of "red apple" much as the collective activity of an ant colony produces an elaborate architectural structure to the colony, although each individual ant may have no appreciation of the overall picture of the nest. There is first the intrinsic information of "red apple."

But how do "I" "know" that I see a red apple? The "red apple" information is bound with the "I" of the above-mentioned "self" circuits. There then is the connection "I-apple" associated with the circuits in the brain. Thus, "I see the apple." *When that bound "I-apple" information becomes associated once more with the information "I" associated with the body map representation in the brain, there is now "I-I-apple" information. Thus, "I recognize that I see the apple," hence consciousness of consciousness.*

Consciousness—Is It Useful?

To more clearly understand why questioning the usefulness of consciousness is inappropriate, instead of asking "What use does consciousness have?", ask "What use does the meaning of the nerve firing patterns of the brain have?" Of course the firing patterns have useful meaning. So consciousness is useful because the firing of the circuits has meaning, which is consciousness itself.

Synesthesia

Synesthesia is a fascinating phenomenon in which certain individuals experience a crossing of sensations (Cytowic, '02; Harrison, '01). Thus, certain people, when looking at numbers or letters, even if the symbols are black, will experience each number or letter as a different specific color. Different synesthetics will differ among themselves as to the actual color of the number or letter. Yet each person retains the same personal experience for his or her lifetime. There are less common examples in which a person may experience music as a particular color, or taste as a particular shape. These experiences can be explained by a cross-wiring of the circuitry. A particular sensory input ends up in a foreign area of the brain. This results in a sensory experience specific for the stimulated brain area, much as stimulating the brain with an electrode will generate a sensory experience specific for that area.

Since different people can experience different primary sensations on examining the same object, one wonders how far such differences actually extend into the full range of human experiences. Are the differing experiences—pleasant, unpleasant, or neutral—that individuals have in viewing art, hearing music, smelling, tasting, or otherwise evaluating situations, based partly on synesthetic-type phenomena? Does one person appreciate a form of esoteric music while regarding much of popular music as noise because of the different arrangement of neuronal circuits, as in synesthesia? Will an artist have little success in selling his painting if the way he views the world differs significantly from the way the population at large sees the world, in a synesthetic sense? Will the public at large appreciate what an artist calls "orange" music if only the artist hears music in that way? Will a pop music star become successful because the artist hears things in the same way that a great many other people do? To what extent are differences in the aesthetic and perceptual senses of individuals the result of congenital neuronal anatomy as opposed to learning? These are as yet unanswered questions worthy of investigation.

Can Zombies Exist?

Is it possible that there could be an individual who acts in all respects like his conscious twin, yet be nonconscious? It is possible that if the person were simply tested with words, as in Searle's Chinese room experiment, then he could fool us into thinking that he was conscious, while not understanding anything that he was saying. Or, he could be in a coma, with his muscles being manipulated like a puppet by an outside source. Then there would still be consciousness, but it would be of the extrinsic variety. The behavior could resemble that of a customarily conscious individual but without customary consciousness. Hence, a *zombie* could exist in that sense, having extrinsic consciousness. Customary consciousness exists, though, if there is intrinsic meaning to the firing circuits, including that of "self" circuits, as well as reportability. If the person has all of these, then the subject is not a zombie, but has customary consciousness, since these are the things that constitute customary consciousness. So a person (or machine) with all the neuronal (or electronic) associations the same as that of a customarily conscious person could not be a zombie.

Consciousness of Additional Spatial Dimensions

Although mathematical equations can easily describe the features of more spatial dimensions than the customary three, we have great difficulty in visualizing four or more spatial dimensions. Is it possible in principle for a brain to be trained to visualize additional spatial dimensions? If the wiring in our brains duplicates the relationships of the outside environment, which we have only seen in three spatial dimensions in evolution and throughout our lives, it is not easy for the brain to contemplate things in more than three spatial dimensions. However, just as the neuronal wiring for seeing in three dimensions could in principle be spread out along two dimensions (in which the nerve cells theoretically are squashed into two dimensions with the same interconnectivity) it should in principle be possible for the right wiring to be set up in the brain to experience more than three spatial dimensions. But the mathematical relations within the circuitry would need to duplicate the kinds of relationships found in mathematical equations involving more than three dimensions.

Consciousness of Higher Levels of Meaning

Consciousness has been presented as the meaning arising from the binding of lower levels of meaning. Is it possible to expand what we experience to yet higher levels of meaning? Submeanings, as described, can combine to produce the quale of red. "Red" and "apple" can go together to produce the image of "red apple." We can from there picture an apple tree, an orchard, etc., building on the levels of organization. At times we can expand further on levels of organization by moments of contemplation, as in visualizing the panorama of a beautiful expanse of mountains. One can then visualize more of the wholeness in the outside world. One may experience feelings of closeness to "God" or, depending on one's world view, a certain unity to the universe and harmony with nature. Such "drawing-in" of diverse information from the environment into the neuronal circuitry can result in higher levels of binding of the information and a higher, more complex, level of consciousness.

How Mind-expansive Can Consciousness Be?

We can be (customarily) conscious of only a very small amount of information at once. Although our brains contain a vast amount of information, only a small amount of it enters the customary conscious mind at a given moment. Can we expand the amount that we are aware of at a given time? Although the Jonah-mind aspect of our brains does have such a broad expanse, the customary part of consciousness does not. According to the thesis presented here, the amount that can enter the customary conscious mind is directly related to the degree that it is reportable at a given time. That is, mechanisms in our brains, for practical purposes, prevent more than a limited amount of information to be in the reportable category at any given time. Without such limitation we would experience chaos and difficulty in taking specific actions in the world because of the myriad of coinciding messages competing for our attention. The brain seems more geared toward the binding of submeanings into higher levels of meaning to achieve a higher complexity of conscious meaning rather than experiencing a multitude of separate conscious meanings at once. With practice, however, people can learn to expand both on the complexity of meaning as well as the number of meanings experienced in a short time.

Seeing with Sound

If customary consciousness is based on intrinsic information in specific areas of the brain, one may well wonder about the situation where a blind patient is fitted with a device that converts light waves into other sensory modality patterns that the patient can eventually learn to experience as "vision." Peter Meijer ('02) has developed a "Soundscapes" device which converts light wave geometric patterns into sound wave patterns that the blind patient can eventually learn to experience as sight, although it is the auditory area of the brain that is directly stimulated. The exciting aspect of this method is that it allows the blind patient to detect the environment significantly away from the body, without having to rely on touch. It would seem then that the information, which is conveyed to the auditory area of the brain, ends up being experienced as visual information. Does this not contradict the idea that stimulation of the auditory area of the brain should give rise to auditory experiences, rather than visual experiences?

The question, though, is whether Soundscapes constitutes actual seeing. Normal people have been doing such an experiment their entire lives in the form of touch. By simply touching an object that is not seen, a person can get some idea of what it looks like. This is not actually vision, even though the person can picture in his or her mind what the touched object might look like. It is more of an *interpretation* of what the object is rather than actual vision. I suspect that this is the kind of experience that the patient who uses "soundscapes" has. Pat Fletcher ('02), a blind woman with significant experience using Soundscapes, has reported that on using the device she can sometimes even sense the sharpness of a pointed object that the soundscapes pattern projects. However, when a normal-seeing patient sees a sharp object, he also can sense that it is likely sharp, without actually feeling the sharpness. So the experience that the blind patient has with Soundscapes may be more of an interpretation than a primary visual experience, much like that of the interpretation resulting from touch.

This is not to deny that under some circumstances the actual structure and function of the auditory area of the brain can be switched to a visual one. In early development, there is greater opportunity for plasticity in the development of structure and function of particular organ systems. For instance, when Sur et al. ('01) cross-wired the sensory input of neonatal ferrets such that visual input ended up in the auditory area of the brain, the latter area developed structure and function suggestive of the visual brain. Both nature, as well as nurture, at the right developmental stages can mold the kinds of circuitry in the brain. Once the structure is established, though, one would expect it would function with specific meaning even if the stimulus were foreign, as by electrode stimulation.

Can a Computer Be Conscious?

Present-day computers to some extent do have reportability and meaning in their circuits. One only has to view the duplication of the environment on a computer screen to see that the numbers within the computer are not simply random and not simply designed to deliver mere word triggers to the outside world. Thus, present-day computers already have a certain degree of consciousness, but with a lot of ambiguity in it, especially when the computer hard disk is separated from its input and output. Computer consciousness is largely extrinsic. When a computer with downloaded music is connected to the environment by loudspeakers, the air waves can transmit the "sound" information to the human eardrum and nervous system. Then, the setup as a whole, which includes the human listener, contains the intrinsic information for sound. If the computer hard drive is considered only in itself, apart from the environment, it still contains the mathematical relationships that distinguish the particular musical selection, but the intrinsic meaning is no longer that of "sound." Extrinsically, the meaning could be music, but it could also be many other things, e.g., a pattern of light waves, if the CD were to be connected to a light transmitter rather than a sound transmitter. Present-day computers, without the human connection, do have a certain degree of customary consciousness, but it is well below the level of human customary consciousness, even when the computer contains a great deal of information about the environment, for following reasons:

1. Present-day computers lack the complex information that is genetically inherited, preformed in the human brain circuitry.
2. Present-day computers are not constructed with the "self" circuits that the human brain has. Thus, the consciousness may be based on intrinsic meaning and be reportable, but is not truly the human variety of customary consciousness, which requires "self" circuits.
3. Despite a great memory for detail about the external environment, computers do not have the tremendous numbers of associations between objects and events in the external world that human beings have. Ever since birth, whenever we take in data from the external environment, we not only register the raw information but relate it to other data that we have acquired, in the Hebbian sense (Hebb, '54), where simultaneously firing neuronal circuits acquire a greater strength of interconnections. This results in a complex of interlocking associations with their emergent properties, and more complex intrinsic information. This massive parallel arrangement of interactive associations differs from the simpler serial sequence of activities that most present-day computers have.

In principle, though, a computer should be able to make such massive parallel interactive associations, and should be able to have "self" circuits (if that were deemed important). This may, in fact, become feasible. Much more difficult, however, would be the creation of computers that have the genetic information that over eons became impressed upon the human brain. We have very little knowledge about the nature of this information, and it would be hard to extract. The mathematics of the brain's information processing is virtually unknown. It is likely, though, that it is based a great deal on associational relationships.

It may be feasible, however, to create conscious computers that have forms of consciousness that differ but are not fundamentally less complex than that of the human brain variety. They might not have the ingrained genetic circuitry or the "self" circuitry, but they could be developed with a high degree of associations among data. Emergent properties of the associations could result in a high level of consciousness that would differ from our own, with the ability to feel events in the environment for which we do not have the proper sensory receptors. In a sense, the Internet is already headed in that direction in view of the increasingly complex interassociations that are part of its structure. Of course, it requires humans at the ends of those associations to interpret the words of the Internet, but when humans are included in the picture, can we look upon the present Internet as having a Mind as a whole?

CHAPTER 15.   THE UNIVERSALITY OF CONSCIOUSNESS

If consciousness = information = meaning, then, since information is everywhere and not just in the brain, one would have to ascribe some degree of consciousness to all areas of the body, indeed everything in the universe. Although *panpsychism* is a common term applied to the idea of consciousness permeating the universe, the type proposed here is very specific. It is not the kind in which the elements of nature have the advanced complexity of human consciousness. There would not be a god of wind and rain and trees with self consciousness, consciousness of consciousness, and myriad attributes associated with the human mind. The complexity of the consciousness would vary with the object, being very simple for a tree or a rock, or a thermostat, so simple as to no longer resemble human consciousness and be difficult, if not impossible, for a human to contemplate.

This viewpoint eliminates the difficulty in trying to explain why consciousness might be attributable to humans and higher animals but never existed through billions of years of evolution of the universe, now suddenly appearing as a new category in an isolated sector of one galaxy among billions. I avoid this problem by proposing that consciousness always existed, everywhere, but at different levels of complexity. This is a difficult concept for many to accept, because we can only be aware of our own consciousness. We presume that other people are also conscious because they look and behave like us, yet the consciousness of others is completely hidden from each of us, let alone the presumed consciousness of non-life forms. It is natural, based on our life experience, which has never experienced any consciousness other than our own, to assume that, apart from other people (or higher animals), consciousness does not exist elsewhere. We rarely stop to consider that consciousness may be everywhere, just as hidden from us as that of other people's conscious experiences, and *we are bathed in a sea of consciousness.*

CHAPTER 16.   CONSCIOUSNESS
IN SPACE AND TIME

If consciousness is meaning, and meaning can arise in a sequence of events that occur over a range of space and time, then consciousness does not simply reflect the events occurring in an instant of time in the brain, but can reflect the meaning of those events over a period of time as well. Thus, in contemplating the picture of a tiger, the information for "tiger" arises during a pattern of neuronal firing that is not only spread out in space, but spread out over time as well. The binding of consciousness into the single picture of "tiger" arises from the meaning of the combined spatial and temporal activity of the brain. Similarly, the meaning of events throughout the universe are spread out over space and time. Therefore, one would also expect that a consciousness ascribed to the universe is not confined to a specific "moment" or "place" but includes that of a broad span of both time and space. Such a bound consciousness, like the proposed human consciousness, would consist of subdivisions, each of which would consist of their own level of consciousness.

CHAPTER 17.   MIND AND THE REAL WORLD—MADE OF THE SAME STUFF?

The preceding discussions explored the concept of consciousness as information, in the form of meaning. This leaves us with more than one kind of thing in the universe. On the one hand, there is Mind, which is information (in the sense of meaning). On the other, there are the objective elements of reality of the external world—matter, space, time, energy. Many physicists consider that all of the latter physical entities—matter, space, time, energy—may one day be fused into a single entity. If that is so, then what about consciousness? Is it something apart from the entities explored by physics, namely just the meaning of physical interactions? Or might consciousness and all of the external world belong to a single category?

Such fusion is conceivable if we regard external reality as pure information and information as consciousness. A simpler way of putting it is to regard the outside world as a "dream." Human consciousness would then be a dream world within a dream world. Human consciousness and all of reality would be made of the same stuff. The dream world of the external world would include, as part of that dream, dream people with dream brains that can duplicate relationships of the primary dream world so as to produce a new dream: that which we call the human mind (or "qualia" or "consciousness") in the sense of this discussion. Just as meaning within the brain results from the associational relationships in the neuronal circuitry, meaning in the outside world would result from similar associational relationships, not necessarily requiring the presence of "objects."

The way the external world could itself *be* information (meaning) is to regard it as a set of relationships among numbers. Science fiction writers discuss the possibility of a universe that is a computer program of which we are unaware. The Platonic idea of a universe that (while not necessarily a program on some giant computer) is the information inherent in a set of relationships among numbers, has some attractive features:

1. There is an aesthetics to the idea, because it fuses consciousness and everything else in the universe into a single entity. If consciousness is based on associations, then perhaps all that external reality requires is associations, such as the mathematical associations of an equation.

2. It becomes easier to view creation, because creation would only require numbers (e.g., the binary numbers zero and one), and all numbers are abstract entities that would seem to be independent of pre-existing space or time for their existence. If equations are also independent of pre-existing space and time, and of necessity exist, and a grand equation for the creation of this universe is one such equation among an infinite number of equations, then this universe could be a self-creating entity in which all the elements stem from numbers and the meaning inherent in one particular set of numbers. A fractal equation (e.g., $z = x + ji$, where i refers to an imaginary number, the square root of minus 1) contains a vast amount of information when laid out as a two-dimensional fractal graphic. There is an infinite number of kinds of equations. Perhaps all varieties of mathematical equations exist, resulting in an infinite number of universes, but we happen to be living in the particular universe that is capable of the formation and development of life.

Since Plato, mathematicians have marveled at the coincidental mathematical relationships that occur throughout nature, which enable the precise description of numerous physical events at the microscopic and macroscopic levels through a few basic equations. It is not so difficult to understand why mathematics is everywhere if we consider the possibility that nature itself may originate from mathematics. We have great difficulty visualizing the concepts of relativity and quantum mechanics. How can space be curved? How can something be a particle and a wave at the same time in quantum mechanics? But despite our difficulty in conceptualizing such things, the math works. The equations of relativity and quantum mechanics are more reflective of reality than the feeble attempts of our minds to picture reality. This may be because the underlying nature of reality is the mathematics itself, rather than the intuitive misconceptions we have about the nature of space and time. Such misconceptions arose from our being confined to only a limited exposure to nature and not experiencing the extremes of space and time, which so shape the laws of quantum mechanics and relativity. Thus our brains did not develop in a way that intuitively could visualize the strange extremes of quantum mechanics and relativity.

When viewing the universe as a whole, we are awestruck by its remarkable complexity and order. Consider, for instance, several key questions about the complexity of the human body:

1. What mechanisms allow it to work in such a magnificent fashion, from the psychological level down to the physiologic and biochemical levels?
2. How did the body ever evolve to such a complex state?
3. What made the laws of nature so precise as to allow the creation of a human body?

Regarding the first question, centuries ago this question would have been answered with the argument that there must be some vitalistic force behind the functioning of the body, for the body is far too complex for a mechanical explanation.

Today, the problem is not problematic philosophically, because we have discovered complex underlying mechanisms that explain the functions of the body.

Regarding the mechanism of evolution of the human body, this is also not so bothersome in principle, since we can postulate genetic selection based on competition and cooperation in nature over many years.

The third question is more problematic than the first two. Even slight variations in the laws of nature (in the relative strengths of the gravitational, electrical and nuclear forces, or in the rate of expansion of the universe) would lead to a universe in which it would be impossible for any sort of life to develop (Gribbin and Rees, '89; Barrow, '02). It is remarkable that the laws are just right so as to permit the presence of life. And it is incredible that relatively few laws of nature can lead to something as remarkable as a human being.

It is an amazing coincidence that relatively small variations of molecular structure can result in biomolecules with totally different functions that fit so precisely into the workings of the body. For instance:

- The complex porphyrin structures of chlorophyll and heme (the oxygen-carrying portion of hemoglobin) differ mainly in the inclusion of an iron molecule in heme and a magnesium ion in chlorophyll. Yet despite the close similarities in structure, the two molecules have very different functions.
- The molecule acetyl CoA is used to provide energy in the Krebs cycle, but is also used as a building block to construct cholesterol, the bile salts, sex hormones, and prostaglandins.
- Glucose may be used to provide energy, or, if it loses a carbon atom, become a structural component of DNA and RNA.
- The sex hormones, cholesterol, chlorophyll, vitamins A, K, and E, and rubber all have a similar substructure consisting of the 5–carbon groupings referred to as isoprenes.
- The amino acids, when necessary, can be converted into carbohydrates or fats.

The biochemical interactions of the body as a whole appear as a vast intertwined network in which variations on a few basic molecular configurations result in molecules with very different functions, which can interact with one another as a seamless, precisely working homeostatic mechanism (Goldberg, '04). Everything fits just right. Is there some compelling reason that the universe had to be precisely as it is, such that it can support life? If not, what (or Who) was responsible for making the laws precisely as they are? Apart from the possibility of a Creator, one could postulate that there has been a succession of universes in which the laws change with each big bang, and we happen to be in the universe in which the laws are just right. However, this would raise the question as to why the laws should change. One could also postulate there are multiple concurrent universes, each of which contains different laws, and we are in that one universe in which the laws are just right. However, considering that our present universe is incredibly vast, it does not seem very economical to postulate an infinite number of other universes just to arrive at an explanation for our own (although this is a possibility).

If, however, one looks at the universe as arising from numbers and numerical relationships, there is no longer a problem with economy. If only numbers are required, that is quite economical. One could postulate an infinite number of grand unified equations for alternate universes, each equation containing a different set of physical constants. Such numbers would not be created, but would exist *of necessity,* numbers being independent of time and space and independent of what anyone or any entity might do. The primary particles and forces would of themselves consist of mathematical relationships. Thus, an infinite set of equations for an infinite set of universes would necessarily exist, and we could then be in one of those universes, one in which the physical laws are just right. This is known as the *anthropic principle,* i.e., that many alternative universes exist, but only one in which the right physical constants exist would allow for people writing and thinking about how the universe originated. That universe is naturally the one in which we would find ourselves.

Our universe would constitute but one meaning that was selected by the anthropic principle from an infinite number of other meanings. With the evolution of the universe, human brains would later come to duplicate the associational relationships of nature, storing information in the form of intrinsic meaning and customary consciousness. Our customary consciousness would be a "dream within a dream." According to this model, *consciousness is the primary structural element of the universe, varying according to the associations within it. Both the universe as well as our minds would be constructed of consciousness.*

How can we say that what we call the "real" world is made of the same stuff as our individual conscious world, when a hurricane in the real world appears so realistic, so different from an imaginary hurricane in our individual conscious world? One reason for this seeming difference is that the real world, of course, would be expected to contain more detail than the fragmentary representations of a hurricane that we conjure up in our minds.

Imagine that a movie is taken of a real hurricane. Imagine that this movie involves advanced technology well beyond that of today, such that the movie is not just in 3-D but contains holographic images of every aspect of the real world down to the molecular level, including all the circuits in a person's brain. The hurricane is now holographic, and so is the holographic person who is interacting with the holographic hurricane. The person in the movie seems to be feeling the brunt of the hurricane, the wind against his body, and a lawn chair that has just struck him in the head. These events are registering in his brain, at least in the imaginary neuronal circuits of his brain that are depicted in the hologram. If consciousness is information, and information does not change when the carrier of the information changes, and the carrier of the original information is now the hologram rather than real molecules, the holographic person should experience consciousness in the same way that a real person would.

Imagine now that the same holographic person just tries to recall his experience in the hurricane. The holographic person will think that the actual hurricane in his external holographic world is real but that his recalled hurricane is merely a thought. He cannot truly feel the brunt of his imagined, recalled hurricane just by recalling it, since the recalled hurricane is not connected to the holographic person's peripheral nerves in a way that would trigger the sensation of the wind or the pain of a chair striking his head. The holographic brain contains only part of the information inherent in the outside holographic world. Although neither the holographic world nor the thoughts of the person in the holographic world are a real world of matter, the holographic external world will seem real to the holographic person, but his own dream world thoughts will not. Thus, the fact that we have completely different impressions about a real hurricane and an imagined hurricane does not mean that our real world could not in itself be a thought.

Another way of looking at this is to ask what information one needs to conceive of "house." One does not have to know what the bricks are composed of, their molecular structure or the quantum mechanical elements that comprise the molecules. A real "house" emerges from the hierarchical structure extending from lower levels of the hierarchy (atoms and molecules) to higher levels (bricks, walls, windows, roof, ceiling etc.). The concept of house still is there, though, even if the lower levels, such as the composition of the bricks, are absent. The difference between a real house and the picture of house in our minds is that the lower levels of the hierarchy are missing in the latter. The full complement of the hierarchy is not there. Human consciousness would then be an incomplete idea within the more complete idea of reality.

CHAPTER 18.   QUANTUM
THEORY AND REALITY

Viewing reality as a thought, as information, provides an easier way to view the particle/wave paradox in quantum theory. In the classic double slit experiment (**Fig. 18–1**), light (or in fact any small particle beam, such as an electron beam) is aimed at a double slit. The resulting pattern on the screen that lies beyond is an interference pattern of the kind indicating some sort of wave interference (**Fig. 18–1B**). The interference pattern would lead one to suppose that such small particles are actually waves, since the interference pattern is best explained by a wave hitting the two slits at once, and then breaking up into two waves, which would then interfere with one another beyond the slits. Even if electrons are aimed one at a time at the double slit, the resulting pattern is an interference pattern. If light or electrons were just particles, then each particle would pass through either of the two slits and give rise to a pattern on the screen that would not have the alternating lines of an interference pattern (**Fig. 18–1A**).

The problem is that in some aspects, light and electrons do appear to act as discrete particles. One dramatic way that this can be seen is in the straight-line track of an electron that travels through an experimental cloud chamber. The particulate nature is also seen in the double slit experiment itself if one uses a screen in which single grains of photographic emulsion deposit when each electron strikes the screen. If a single electron is allowed to pass through the slit apparatus and strikes the screen, what appears is a solitary dot of developed emulsion on the screen, rather than a diffuse pattern of developed silver grains. As each successive electron reaches the screen, more and more dots form on the screen, until a final pattern arises. The final pattern, though, is an interference pattern, the same pattern that would occur on aiming many electrons at once through the two slits. The interference pattern suggests waves.

The paradox in the wave-particle controversy, then, is that on the one hand the electron appears to be a particle (individual dots on the screen). On the other hand, the electron appears to be a wave (the interference pattern).

How can something be both a particle and a wave at the same time? One way of approaching this dilemma is to ignore it, just focusing on the practicality of the mathematical applications of quantum theory. If the math works and can predict

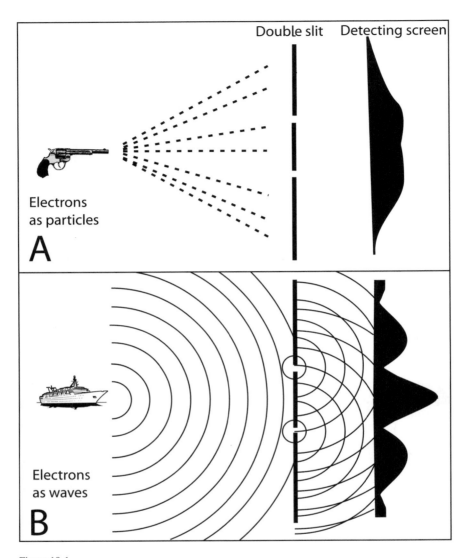

Figure 18-1

what will be observed, then that is all that we need to talk about, and we can't understand the underlying reality. The reality may be akin to the blind men feeling the elephant. One feels the tail and the other feels the trunk. Each comes to a different conclusion as to what an elephant is. Or consider the analogy with the classic vase/profile illusion (**Fig. 18–2**). Is it a vase or two facial profiles? Imagine two people going into a room to observe this figure. One comes out saying that she saw faces while the other says he saw a vase. If we have never seen the figure but rely only on the reports of the two observers, we would have great difficulty in under-

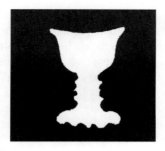

Figure 18-2

standing how two people looking at the same thing could see such different things. Perhaps the wave/particle controversy is of such a nature. Things depend on how we observe them.

The Heisenberg uncertainty principle regards the wave quality of the electron as an uncertainty as to its position. The uncertainty lies not just in one's ignorance of the position of a particle that in reality has a clear-cut position. The reality is that it has no clear-cut position, only a probable position. It is, in a sense, in many places at once, spread out as a "probability wave" that can interact with other probability waves and generate interference patterns. According to one explanation, when the wave encounters a measuring device and a particle is detected, the wave collapses to form a localized particle, such as a silver grain on the screen in the double-slit experiment. It is unpredictable, even in principle, whether the particle will appear on the left or the right side of the screen. If there is a "collapse of the wave function," it remains a question as to precisely when the collapse occurs and what qualities a measuring apparatus needs to have to cause the collapse. Why should the uncertainty surrounding the electron's position not be transmitted to the screen and to all future events involving the screen or any other measuring device?

One theory is that the electron is always a particle, but is accompanied by a separate probability wave that determines its position. This theory (developed by Bohm) is not popular, in part because it requires the postulation of two separate things: a particle and a separate coinciding wave.

The *Many-Worlds Theory* (Bruce, '04) avoids the collapse of the wave by assuming that the electron is a particle that exists simultaneously in many worlds, in a different position in each world, and that these worlds interact to produce the interference pattern. Each of the worlds also has a copy of ourselves viewing a different position of the particle on the screen in each world. An objection to the Many-Worlds Theory is that it is not very economical on worlds.

Some authors have suggested that human consciousness has a unique mysterious quality that collapses the wave, i.e., that only the act of human conscious observation causes the collapse (Goswami, '93). The interpretation that requires human consciousness to create reality leads to the paradox know as "Schroedinger's Cat." Irwin Schroedinger, one of the founders of quantum mechanics, imagined a live cat inside a closed box. A quantum decision, namely, whether or not a particular quantum particle will undergo radioactive decay, is about to happen in the box. If the decay occurs, this will set into action a device that will kill the cat. If the decay does not occur, then the cat lives. Does the cat die or not? One does not know until the box is opened. If the reality of the decay depends on the human observation, then the reality of whether or not the cat is alive (which is a macroscopic, not just a quantum, event) is not set until the box is opened. One could not say that some decision as to the cat's fate was already determined prior to opening the box. In quantum mechanics, the indeterminacy of the cat's status is not just the practical one of not knowing what actually happened before the box is opened. There supposedly would be no reality to either the cat's being alive or dead until the box is opened and the cat observed, since there is no reality of the quantum event until the box is opened for the person to observe. Thus, indeterminacy at the quantum level would be extended into the macroscopic realm, and reality would depend on one's conscious observation. However, the problem with this reasoning, insofar as consciousness is concerned, is that one can readily imagine a human observer actually opening the box and seeing what the cat's status is. One would presume that this brought the reality of the situation into existence. But what if that observer were himself in a still larger box that encompassed everything, and a second observer had to open that larger box to find out what the first observer had experienced? Then, from the point of view of the second observer, the event would be indeterminate until he opened that larger box. Events would be indeterminate even though a human observer (the first observer) had already been consciously involved with the observation. Or do we say that only the first contact with a conscious being is critical in the collapse of the wave? The physicist John Bell ('90) has remarked "What exactly qualifies some physical systems to play the role of 'measurer'? Was the wave function of the world waiting to jump for thousands of years until a single-celled living creature appeared? Or did it have to wait a little longer, for some better qualified system . . . with a PhD?"

What gives something the quality of being a "measurer"? The thesis of this book does not support the hypothesis that *only* human beings can cause the "collapse of the wave function" through the act of human observation. Consciousness (information) is everywhere. Why should only the particular consciousness of human beings have this unique ability? Human beings, like inanimate matter, are composed of molecules. Why should one set of molecules be able to cause the collapse but not another? The idea that only humans can do it is perhaps a throwback to the need by some to postulate an anthropocentric universe. It is likely that "collapse" of the wave function (or the splitting into many worlds in the Many-Worlds hypothesis) can occur at many places apart from the human brain. Penrose (Folger, '05) has suggested that the collapse occurs when the wave interacts with matter that exceeds a certain minimal mass and gravity.

The interpretations of the wave/particle controversy present many conceptual difficulties. It is hard to visualize what is meant by a probability wave, by a collapse of such a wave, a wave/particle, or a positioning of an electron in many worlds that interact with one another. However, by viewing reality as a dream, as consciousness, as information, it becomes a bit easier to picture this situation, as follows:

Consider the sound "hee," which we mentioned means "he" in English but "she" in Hebrew. Imagine the word registering in the brain of an observer who understands both English and Hebrew. What does the word mean prior to the person's translating it? On the one hand, we could say it means nothing since it is only an untranslated word that will trigger brain events that will give rise to an interpretation. The word does not in itself contain intrinsic information as to sex. On the other hand, we could say it has extrinsic information for both "he" and "she" in respect to the two different language-translating mechanisms. We have little difficulty in understanding how a word could be ambiguous since it is only a word, which under one circumstance could mean one thing and under another circumstance mean something else. However, suppose that instead of a word, we were to look at a real person who was heavily clothed in a way that we could not determine at a glance whether the person was male or female. We would say that we did not know the person's sex, but without a doubt the sex had to be either male or female. It could not conceivably be both, as could the sound "hee." We can accept an ambiguity in the word, but not in the actual physical person.

Something of this nature may relate to the difficulty in comprehending the reality of the wave/particle in quantum theory. If we regard the electron as a real physical object, like the person in clothes, then we cannot see how it could simultaneously be both a particle and a wave. However, if we regard the electron as we do the word, as information that is ambiguous in meaning, not as yet fully defined, as existing in a probabilistic equation, then it is easier to view how it could be a particle and a wave at the same time. Thus, reality is not one of physical objects, but of information, of meaning. If there is a wave collapse, it is a situation wherein the information is interpreted, as the word "hee" is interpreted to mean "he" or "she." If there is no collapse (the Many-Worlds Theory) then rather than dealing with the lack of economy of a "Many-Worlds" theory, there is the economy of a "Many-Meanings" theory. If the sound "hee" remains untranslated, it could be interpreted as meaning both "he" and "she" or, for that matter, an infinite number of other things. Similarly, in the Many-Worlds Theory, the position of the particle would remain undefined (albeit mathematically undefined), and the particle would have the meanings of existing in many locations at once.

Rather than using quantum mechanics to understand consciousness (see the discussion on quantum mechanics and the Binding Problem in Chapter 14), it may be more useful to use consciousness to understand the paradoxes of the quantum world.

CHAPTER 19.   FREE WILL,
GOD, AND THE SOUL

The idea of free will is central not only to religion but to the legal system, which holds people responsible for their actions. If free will exists, then one's actions have an aspect that is nondeterministic. Whereas in the nineteenth century nondeterministic mechanisms would have been deemed impossible from a scientific standpoint, the advent of quantum mechanics has allowed for indeterminism. A common example of a quantum mechanical "decision" is radioactive half-life. Radioactive substances decay at certain rates, which vary according to the specific kinds of atoms that are undergoing decay. Each clustering of radioactive atoms has a certain half-life, the time in which half of the atoms will decay. According to quantum theory, the decision as to which atom will decay does not depend on hidden variables that distinguish one atom from another. It is an intrinsic quality of matter that within a given span of time half of the atoms will decay and half will not, even if all the atoms are subject to precisely the same conditions. One cannot even in principle predict which atom will decay. The event is indeterminate.

Another classic example of nondeterminism in quantum mechanics is the double slit experiment, described in Chapter 18. The interference pattern on the screen suggests wave interference, but the deposition of individual dots on the screen suggests particles and that the photon wave suddenly "collapses" into a single spot when striking the screen. The exact location of the spot of a given collapse (e.g., to the left or right side of the screen) cannot be predicted even in principle.

Quantum mechanics regards the selection of the atom that will decay radioactively as completely random. One may well ask what this has to do with free will. If a so-called free will decision is indeterminate in the quantum sense, how can you call it free will if it is based on randomness? A neuron may or may not fire, based on the sum total of stimulatory and inhibitory synaptic input. If that decision is influenced one way or the other by quantum mechanics, and that decision is random, then there still is no basis for free will.

However, the concept of randomness needs further clarification. Can one truly say that anything is random (Pagels, '82)? The number 6920443710819621278638824 appears random and may in fact have been generated by some random process. However, suppose that in the next room there is a number 80315548219307323897499935, which also was randomly generated. The first number subtracted from the second gives 11111111111111111, hardly a random number. Suppose there are other rooms, each of which contains randomly generated numbers, but which also result in differences consisting of orderly patterns. The individual numbers may be randomly generated, but the relationships between them imply an order that is not random.

As a visual example, consider the random dot stereogram (**Fig. 19–1**). The dots in the left box are completely randomly placed, as are those on the right. However, when viewed in stereo (try looking straight in the distance through the figures), a square appears in the background. That is because a small segment in the left box in the form of a square has been displaced slightly to one side, still leaving a random pattern, but one that differs from the right box by the dislocation of one square patch of dots.

The point is that individual atomic events may be random, but the relationships between them may not be. Thus, if one considers the numerous synaptic firings that

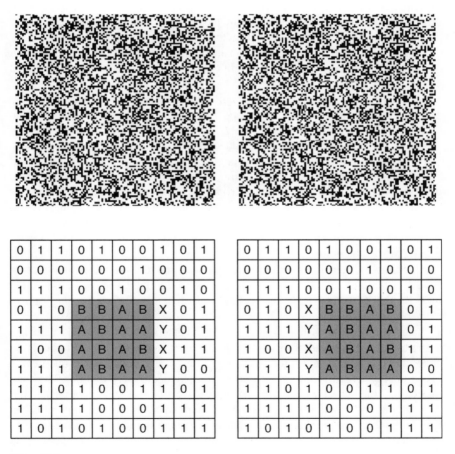

Figure 19-1

must occur during a thought, the quantum events that may decide the firing or not firing of an individual neuron may be random in the true sense of quantum theory. However, the collective effect of the relationships of all the synaptic firings together could present with something that is not random. Could this provide a basis for free will, an indeterminism not based on randomness? The collective firings, the relationships of activity between the firing neurons during a single thought, constitute an emergent, bound property, that of information, that of meaning, as a single functioning whole. Could information (consciousness) then in some way result in a free will decision, even though the individual quantum events are random? The self is information in the brain. Could the self make indeterminate decisions that are nonrandom while staying within the rules of quantum theory?

Even if decisions were found to be purely random, is it still possible that randomness can be the basis for free will? For instance, in the slit screen experiment, the decision as to whether the particle will fall to the right or left is regarded as completely random. What if this choice results in a life-or-death result, depending on whether the particle landed right or left? Could something steer the overall effect of many quantum decisions toward a particular critical outcome (or striking "coincidence") while still falling within the realm of quantum randomness?

All this, of course, is pure speculation and is simply presented to discuss the *potentiality* for free will within the realm of quantum mechanics, without showing a compelling scientific reason for it.

A difficulty in using quantum mechanics as an explanation for free will is the problem of how this would really work. If we reject the dualistic proposal that there is a separate mind outside the body, how could a free will decision, particularly a moralistic one, be made without an outside mind? Any decision would have to be based on the existing neuronal circuitry rather than a mystic mind. What would enable this circuitry to have a "mind of its own" that could direct free will decisions (Churchland, '02)? Moreover, one would expect even the Jonah-minds of the brain to exhibit their own free will decisions, something beyond the control of the areas of the brain involved in customary consciousness. Should we hold the individual responsible for decisions made by the so-called "unconscious" (Jonah-mind) parts of the brain?

Alternatively, there is no such thing as free will, and it only appears to us that we have it. In that case, making a so-called personal free will decision involves nothing more than the firing of "self" circuits along with other information-carrying circuits in the brain. The events of such firing are undoubtedly extremely complex, so much so that it would be impossible to predict in practical terms what decision a person is going to make despite all efforts to obtain the information that the brain holds. In chaos theory, the so-called "butterfly effect" refers to the great changes in outcome in complex systems that may arise from even the slightest of perturbations. The brain may exhibit the butterfly effect when making a decision that we cannot predict, but even so, this still would imply a type of determinism, at least in principle. It is just that the system is too complex for anyone to fully understand all the details.

If there is no free will, what basis can we have for punishing wrongdoing? Is punishment then fair to the perpetrator? Although it is possible that punishment may serve to detract others from committing crimes, a more valid reason for punishment is that it may discourage the individual from committing further crimes. And if this is not effective, at least the person, through imprisonment or other institutionalization, would not be in a position to repeat the behavior. It may serve society's interests to act "as if" there were free will, even it it doesn't exist. It would be important though to distinguish those acts that are beyond the person's control from those that the person can conceivably control. For instance, if the individual commits a crime while having an attack of temporal lobe epilepsy, that is not controllable, so there would be less justification for punishment. However, if it is deemed possible that the person could have prevented the behavior, then punishment would make more sense. The difficulty in the legal process lies in knowing whether or not the behavior is controllable. For an excellent in-depth discussion of free will and morality from a scientific standpoint, see Shermer ('04).

God and the Soul

Thus far in the book, the questions of the existence of God and the soul have not been discussed. Does God exist? This is really not a good question. In a sense, depending on how one defines God, everyone believes in God, even atheists. To one person God is the unifying equation for the universe, coming into existence with the universe without creating it. The universe is in this view self-creating. To others, the universe was self-creating and also has a Mind. To another, God is the creator of the universe, but no longer participates in it after the original creation. To others, God is creator and continues to influence the course of the universe in the form of the rules of nature, without the introduction of miracles. To others there is a Creator God who participates in the course of the universe, and may use miracles, events beyond the realm of natural law. And to many others, the concept of God is accompanied by complex customs and beliefs, often contradictory among the various religions, about what God wants of humans and what people should do in this world. And to many, religion includes the existence of an immortal Soul.

This book has presented reasons for considering human consciousness (the "mind") as being equivalent to information in the brain. There does not appear to be evidence that there is something else, namely a Soul that differs from consciousness itself. This does not mean, however, that there may not be an immortality associated with the mind, a topic to be discussed below. It seems simplest to equate the mind with the soul, rather than introducing a second conscious entity.

If consciousness is information, and there is a vast amount of information outside the human brain, then this thesis proposes that there is a consciousness, or Mind, associated with the universe, which might even be infinite. It would appear unnecessary to propose the presence of a God as an entity separate from the Mind of the universe.

If humans have free will, it would be reasonable to ask whether there is free will to the Mind of the universe (i.e., a Mind that can interact with the universe), since the human mind and Mind of the universe both consist of information, although at vastly different levels of organization. Now one may object that there cannot possibly be an influence of such a universal Mind on the workings of the universe since the structure of the universe is so different from that of the human body. Objects in the universe are so disconnected at far distances from one another, whereas the human body contains a rich interconnection of parts, particularly the nervous system, which enables communication between one area of the body and another. However, recalling our problem (in the beginning of this chapter) about how quantum mechanical decisions could be the basis for free will when quantum mechanical decisions are random, it was pointed out that while two (or more) quantum mechanical systems may be making random decisions, the correlations between the systems might not be random. According to quantum mechanics, such correlation can be a *nonlocal* action, i.e., one that does not necessarily depend on direct communication between the systems. Such nonlocal, "entangled" correlations are strongly founded in quantum mechanics (Mermin, '85).

Thus, it is conceivable that there could be instantaneous nonrandom decisions involving very distant aspects of the universe. They are not the sort of decisions where one element of the universe can instantly affect a distant area by sending useful information from one area to another. That is the mistaken claim of parapsychology, which to the author's knowledge, still has no convincing basis (Blackmore, '04), and is a form of communication that is not allowed by quantum mechanics. Rather, the interaction in quantum mechanics is that of a nonrandom correspondence between distant random events instead of a transmission of information from one place to another. It is sort of like each piece of the random-dot stereogram (**Fig. 19–1**) being in a different location in the universe. Having access to only one of the pieces cannot provide the picture of the recessed square. The correlation between the two random-dot pieces is still there though. Suppose the patterns on the two pictures are constantly changing, such that they always represent individually random configurations, but yet are always correlated with one another. That is, the change of pattern in picture A is always correlated with a slightly shifted pattern in picture B to represent, for example, a triangle, circle, or square as the difference. Neither the observer at A nor the observer at B would know about the triangle, circle, or square, but the information would still exist in an entangled way. It is a type of action at a distance, but one that does not allow relaying of specific information from observer A to observer B. Can we can rule out such type of nonrandomness as part of the workings of the universe?

Parapsychology

Parapsychology asks whether one individual can be aware of another's thoughts at a distance, where the two have no possibility of communicating in the customary sense. While this book proposes that there is a hierarchical binding of all activity in the universe, there is no reason to suppose that lower levels of the hierarchy can "know about" or influence higher levels or other members at the same level. One would expect that binding between one individual's mind and that of others would be in the form of a Jonah-mind, extrinsic information that is not reportable. Whether a higher level can influence a lower level is an interesting question, but that in effect is the free will issue of whether God (or lower levels of the Universe hierarchy – "angels"?) can exert an influence, whether in the form of "miracles" or natural coincidences. One would like to feel that this is the case, but is there any hard evidence for it?

Immortality

The human species has undergone a series of blows to its ego. Centuries ago scientists challenged the idea that the earth was the center of the universe. It became clear that the earth revolves around the sun, not the opposite, and our sun is but one sun of billions in our galaxy, among billions of galaxies. It made us feel rather small. The theory of evolution did not help, telling us that we descended from apes and contain 99% of ape DNA along with many ape mannerisms.

Vitalism has retreated since the 19th century. There is no longer a vital substance, a mystical spark of life, that is breathed into an otherwise inanimate body. Life is the result of the complex processing that occurs in the body from the macroscopic levels of anatomy and physiology to microscopic levels of cell biology, biochemistry, and biophysics.

The remaining bastion of the human ego is consciousness. The dualistic viewpoint regards consciousness as a mysterious entity, separate from the body just as vitalism separated a life force from the body. Some people call consciousness the "Soul," something that is believed by many to have an associated immortality. Consciousness has been regarded as a late development in evolution, something peculiar to man and which separates man from other forms of life and certainly from inanimate matter. However, the point of view in this book, that consciousness is information (meaning), removes the mystical element from consciousness and even appears to further reduce our uniqueness in the universe. Since information is not unique to human beings, consciousness is everywhere and has existed since the beginning of the universe, wherever there is information. If the mind is information is there any need to postulate something different, a "Soul"?

The "Soul" may be none other than consciousness. Shouldn't this disappear, like the body, when the brain dies? Although claims have been made for a Soul and an afterlife based on near-death experiences, the interpretations of such experiences have been very much open to criticism, particularly that they may simply represent normal physiological reactions of the body and altered mental states at the time of certain great bodily stresses (Blackmore, '04). If there is no afterlife, what then is there for a human being to be proud of, having descended from apes on a planet lost in a myriad of galaxies, with a life and consciousness explainable in terms of cheap chemicals and ordinary information, whose only end is permanent death?

In reality, the situation is quite the opposite. Equating consciousness with information can lead to a far more inspiring viewpoint than a dualistic view of consciousness that is based on metaphor and mysticism. Equating consciousness with information provides a logical and inspirational way of approaching the question of our relation to the universe and to "God" and the question of immortality. If consciousness is information, then what can we say of all the information in the universe? It, too, must have an emergent quality, which one could refer to, on this larger scale, as the Mind of God. If our universe is infinite (or if there are infinite other universes), then the Mind of God is infinite, too. *If* we have free will (no conclusion was arrived at in this book), then the larger emergent quality of all the information in the universe may also have free will, since it is made of the same stuff, only at a higher level. The Mind of God could then interact with the universe rather than remain the silent observer of a once-created universe.

The Spinozan view of God *being* nature, or in this case *being* the information in the universe, as opposed to preceding the universe and creating the universe, has for many centuries been a point of philosophical and religious dispute, but it need not be. The points of view are really rather close. The idea of God's preceding and then creating a universe supposes that time pre-existed the universe, in order to allow a God the opportunity to accomplish the creation. From a religious perspective, it is unacceptable to think in terms of God originating *with* the universe if time and a spatial void existed before the universe was created, thereby preceding God. However, if the origin of the universe included the first appearance not only of matter, but also of space and time, then *nothing* preceded the origin of the universe. God, then would have existed since the beginning of time.

The idea of humans evolving from apes should not degrade our status. What we have evolved *into* is vastly more complex and can accomplish far more than an ape can. Emergent properties combine with emergent properties to produce higher-level emergent properties, which are qualitatively quite different from the quantitative sum of their parts. It is not one's origin that counts towards a person's value. It is what the person becomes, what the person does with his/her life that counts.

Equating consciousness with information also has something to say about immortality. Rather than the mythical resurrection of decayed bodies and skeletons that will somehow emerge from the grave with new life, there is a logical immortality that can occur through information. Since information can present in different formats, the information that constitutes a person could, in principle, be preserved without the body. The idea of storing a person's mind in computer format is presently the stuff of science fiction. While it may be possible in principle, it would require a technology far more advanced than anything available today to extract not only the thoughts, but the memories and information processing mechanisms in a brain. Moreover, it would require not only tapping a person's customary consciousness, but the totality of Jonah-minds which, together with customary consciousness, might be considered a "Soul."

Immortality, however, can be approached by a different means. Consider a piece of black paper. It is not just a piece of black paper, but in a way contains all the information in the universe written in black pen on a white paper until the paper eventually becomes black. The black paper in a sense contains infinite information, including the information that would constitute one's mind. Does a wooden block contain no meanings within it, or does it contain an infinite number of sculptures, an infinite number of persons, an infinite number of meanings? Such infinite information, which would exist at all places and times, would include that of a person's mind. Thus one's Soul, or Mind, when looked at in this manner, has been around forever, and will persist for all time in all parts of the universe. Resurrection is thus ever-existing.

The equation of consciousness with information provides a contemporary view of the Mind and God. It has nothing to say one way or the other about the rituals and customs of present religions. It merely provides a more reasoned framework of thinking about the Mind, God, and immortality, one that could fit in just as well with the other tenets of the various religions.

CHAPTER 20.   THE FUTURE

This book, while discussing consciousness as a function of the brain, has not gone into much neuroanatomy, physiology, or biochemistry. To what degree can studies in these fields contribute to an understanding of the "hard" problem of consciousness, i.e., why consciousness should arise during activity in the brain?

There are some who feel that such studies will contribute little, since the "hard" problem of consciousness is subjective and not likely to be resolved with the objective techniques of science, or at best may only be approached by introspection. Others feel strongly that scientific research can eventually solve the problem.

I maintain an intermediary point of view. The proposal in this book is that consciousness arises from the duplication of the associative relationships in nature. One can in principle explore this by further study of the patterns of interneuronal connections ("neuronal nets"), a difficult area of study which nonetheless is making steady progress (Churchland PS, '02; Churchland PM, '95; Spitzer, '99). The question is whether, in the end, studies will confirm the idea that the patterns of connection in the nervous system are in fact organized according to associative relationships that duplicate those of the environment.

Introspection already provides strong clues that the nervous system acts through associative relationships. I see this every morning when doing the word scramble puzzle in the newspaper. As part of the puzzle, one needs to unscramble the letters and determine what word is represented by, e.g., "oginrwc." In a serial computer, the approach would be to try all different combinations of the letters and then match the resulting words with a dictionary to determine if any of the words were actual English words. The person, though, can arrive at the answer by first noting that the letters "ing" are commonly found in words. Considering the category of "ing," what words would have the remaining letters "orwc" in them along with "ing" at the end? This narrows the search and enables one to quickly determine that the word is "crowing." We associate virtually everything. Mention "red," and there immediately comes to mind "apple," "rose," "catsup," "blood," "red hair," "fire," etc., and each of these words will call to mind a long list of other words that relate to those categories. The brain houses a complex web of neuronal interactions. We do have associative minds. Neurophysiological studies could help confirm this and show the physical structure of those associations.

We already have some inroads into the mechanism of associations and categories. In the visual system, in particular, it has been shown that there is a hierarchical organization such that particular patterns of information from the retina stimulate "simple" cells in the visual cortex, and patterns of information coming from simple cells stimulate "complex" cells in the brain. For instance, a simple visual cortical cell might respond only to a straight line lying at a particular angle and moving in a particular direction on the retina. Then there are "complex" cells that require a pattern of firing of simple cells in order to fire them. Hence, there is the idea of a complex "grandmother" cell that responds only to the visual information of "grandmother." It can be seen that the association of groups of simple and complex cells in forward and backward feedback loops can provide a possible framework for the associative nature of human thought and the duplication of the associative relationships of the environment. For example, in the discussion above regarding the word scramble puzzle, there may be "ing" cells that when stimulated provide feedback loops to the numerous words that end in "ing."

A key reason for the difficulty in determining the structural relationships within neuronal nets is that different anatomical patterns can, in principle, give rise to the same general associational relationships. No two nervous systems are wired the same anatomically, just as no two faces are exactly alike. Even if two brains had an identical thought, the exact anatomy of neuronal connections for the thought is unlikely to be the same in the two brains. It is like the situation in the opening break of a game of pool. If one looks at the resulting lie of the balls when their motion stops, there would be few, maybe even only one, pattern in which all the balls could have been positioned in the opening break to arrive at such a final lie. However, at the time of the break it is not possible to predict the exact position of all the balls at the end even if you tried your best to examine the precise angle and speed of the balls at the break. Slight variations in the angle and speed of the white ball, or quantum mechanical fluctuations could result in a multitude of different final patterns even though the initial break looked the same in all cases. The same initial break, then could result in a multitude of final lies on the table, each of which corresponded to only one specific initial break. In the nervous system as well, a multitude of variations on the neuronal net patterns in the brain could correspond to the same conscious experience, so long as the net associations among the elements of the net are similar (**Fig. 20–1** and **20–2**). In **Figs. 20–1** and **20–2** the numbered circles refer to nerve cells, the arrows to neuronal connections. Both of these figures have different anatomical layouts but indentical patterns of connective associations.

All faces have eyes, nose, mouth, and ears, but they are put together in somewhat different ways in different individuals. We would need to find the "eyes, nose, mouth, and ears" of the neuronal interconnections, the actual associational relationships, not an easy task. The value of such studies, if they are eventually successful, is that one then might be able to dissect a conscious experience such as "red" into its subcomponents, which remain hidden as Jonah-minds, and we may ultimately come to a better understanding of the true roots of consciousness and the "hard" problem.

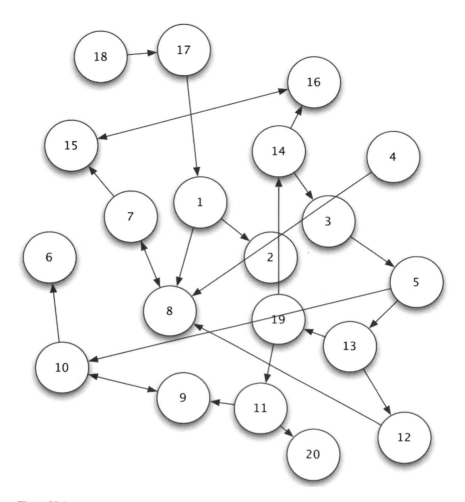

Figure 20-1

In order to maintain the focus of our conscious thoughts on a single idea, a mechanism is required that operates at a more macroscopic level to enable such focusing to occur, instead of widespread wild firing of all circuits at once. Studies at a higher level of brain organization (Edelman et al., '02) may help to determine how this comes about, how we can maintain consciousness of one thing at a time and not be overwhelmed by everything at once. Such studies are misdirected, however, if they aim to find out how consciousness per se arises. As discussed in Chapter 4, it is a fallacy to believe that there are some areas of the nervous system that are conscious and others that are not, and that by examining the difference between these areas, one will find the mysterious roots of what consciousness is. As

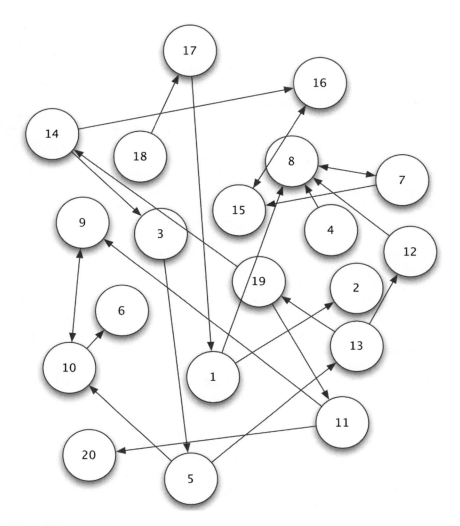

Figure 20-2

discussed, the difference between the conscious and so-called unconscious areas of the nervous system is not that one area is conscious and the other not. All areas are conscious. It is just that one area is capable of reporting on its consciousness, while the other cannot and is a Jonah-in-the-whale, a Jonah-mind. Studies at the gross level of organization may provide information as to how the nervous system provides reportability versus nonreportability, but are not likely to shed light on the true nature of consciousness, which is a more universal entity, not even confined to the brain or to organic matter.

Future Social Issues

If a computer can be conscious, this raises certain ethical issues in dealing with future computer-based consciousness. It is not known if it ever will be possible to duplicate a person's conscious thought processes and place them in computerized format, or to do the reverse, directly transfer to the brain a computerized thought, much like a Macintosh program might be converted to a Windows-compatible format. If consciousness reduces in the end to mathematical relationships, then it should be possible in principle to do these things, even though it might never be practicable. Knowledge of the synaptic connections within the human brain is only about a hundred years old, and reasonably complex computers have existed for only about half that time. Given the pace of scientific advances, one can only speculate on how complex computers might become within several hundred years, and whether mind-to-computer or computer-to-mind transfers may be feasible. If they are, then certain issues will surely arise:

Imagine an advanced society that is overwhelmed with information. There is too much to know and too little time to learn it. Research eventually finds a way to directly hook up the computerized information of the world with the brain to allow instant access to the world's information without the tedium of current searches. Further advances permit the reverse, the transfer of human thoughts to a computer.

- If one can transfer a human mind to a computer format, could this be used as a means of achieving immortality? Could a person elect to transfer his mind to a computer, and then have someone kill his sick and aging biological body to avoid the anguish of prolonged death? Would such a killing be immoral, or even considered a true death, for, after all, the mind would still persist, albeit in computerized format? Which is more important to preserve, the mind or the body?
- If one's mind were transferred to a computer, could one destroy the computer representation of the mind, or would this be considered an act of murder?
- If one were to duplicate the mind, much like one makes a copy of a computer program, would one be justified in later destroying one of the copies, or would each copy be considered a separate life, which must be preserved?
- If a computer were developed with a program so complex that it approached the complexity of a human brain, would there be some point at which one would say that there is a consciousness to this computer that is complex enough as to make it wrong to terminate it, much as it would be wrong to terminate a human life?
- Why do we feel it wrong to allow people to kill one another? Is it because it is intrinsically wrong to do so, or, for practical reasons, because it would lead to malfunctioning of society, to widespread fighting and discontent, so the laws have to be protective of life, by common agreement? If it is intrinsically wrong to kill for religious/moralistic reasons, then perhaps it would be wrong to kill an artificially developed computer mind, unless one believed that a computer-mind could not in any way be given the same kind of respect that a human mind deserves. If it is wrong to kill for practical reasons, then per-

haps there would be nothing wrong with terminating defenseless conscious computers, which would be incapable of fighting back and harming people.

Such issues are very remote from the present state of computers, but conceivably could be issues in the far distant future. A more reasonable prediction for the future is the prospect of the development of an extremely intelligent computer that duplicates much of the abilities of the human brain and can learn as it develops, just as a child learns from birth. Would it then be feasible to raise computer children as if they were our own offspring, children who could achieve immortality?

CHAPTER 21.   SUMMARY

This book attempts to resolve the "hard" problem of consciousness, namely how consciousness can arise from the brain. The proposal is dualistic. Namely, there are the brain and the information it contains. Consciousness is information. Much of the book is involved with the definition of information and how it can arise in the brain.

Chapter 1 (THE DEFINITION OF CONSCIOUSNESS AND THE MIND/BODY PROBLEM) begins by defining consciousness as the experiences we have, such as "red," "smell of rose," "taste of coffee," "sound of a horn," "light touch," "pain," the emotions and all manner of thoughts that seem so different from the actual structure of the brain, with which consciousness is associated.

Chapter 2 (THE IMPORTANCE OF THE MIND/BODY PROBLEM) summarizes key questions associated with the topic of consciousness and why those topics are important to address.

Chapter 3 (THE ORIGIN OF OF CONSCIOUSNESS—CURRENT THEORIES) reviews current theories of consciousness including dualism, monistic materialism, and monistic idealism, as well as their difficulties.

Chapter 4 (TOWARD A NEW THEORY OF CONSCIOUSNESS) makes three proposals toward a new theory of consciousness:

1. Consciousness is information. Thus there is a Brain and the information within it, accounting for the "Brain/Mind" duality.
2. Consciousness comes in a broad spectrum, from simple to complex.
3. All areas of the brain are conscious. That is, it may be that those brain areas that are traditionally called unconscious are actually conscious but hidden from us in the same way that another person's consciousness is hidden from us.

I introduce the term "Jonah-mind" to indicate the hidden nature of this consciousness, just as Jonah is a conscious being in the (hypothetically intelligent, verbal) whale, which does not experience Jonah's thoughts and cannot report on it to others. I caution the reader not to consider a Jonah-mind as a little person inside the brain. The Jonah-mind can represent any level of consciousness, even the most miniscule, without a sense of "self" or other higher levels of complexity.

We thus have our "customary" consciousness, which we can report on to others, and our pockets of "Jonah-mind" consciousness, which we cannot.

Chapter 5 (CONSCIOUSNESS = INFORMATION = MEANING) defines "information" as used in this book. By "information" I do not use the quantitative definition of information as applied in information theory, but the more qualitative definition of "meaning," namely what something refers to.

Chapter 6 (FORMATS, CARRIERS, AND TRIGGERS OF INFORMATION) cautions the reader not to confuse information in the brain with formats of information (e.g., the kind of code used to transmit information), carriers of information (e.g., brain tissue itself), or triggers of information (e.g., a pin-prick as opposed to the sensation that it triggers).

Chapter 7 (INTRINSIC VERSUS EXTRINSIC MEANING IN CONSCIOUSNESS) explains that meaning can be intrinsic or extrinsic. Intrinsic meanings are obvious from examining relationships within the object itself. Extrinsic meanings are relationships outside the object. For instance, a circle has the intrinsic meaning of an unending path arising from the set of all points equidistant from a central point. A word, though, has only extrinsic meaning, being meaningless in itself except in reference to an outside dictionary. A human observer is not necessary for meaning to arise.

Chapter 8 (CUSTOMARY CONSCIOUSNESS IN PART REQUIRES REPORTABLE INTRINSIC MEANING) shows that the meaning (information) associated with customary consciousness in our brains is an intrinsic meaning, since any extrinsic meaning would be a Jonah-mind and nonreportable. In order for that intrinsic meaning to constitute customary consciousness, as opposed to just a Jonah-mind consciousness, it needs to be reportable by the person to the outside world.

Chapter 9 (HOW THE FIRING OF BRAIN CIRCUITS CAN HAVE INTRINSIC MEANING) shows how consciousness can arise in the brain as a duplication of the associational relationships found in the world in space and time. Rather than the firing patterns of neurons being some kind of code that needs to be translated, the firings are an actual duplication of world events in the form of associational relationships. It is the meaning of the associational relationships that constitutes consciousness.

The proposal in this book that consciousness is information should not be categorized as a form of "functionalism." In functionalism, consciousness depends on what function is ascribed to the information processing in the brain, how the brain interacts with its environment. In this book's proposal, such function is unnecessary. Consciousness would exist even if the brain were preserved in a vat with no communication with the outside world.

Chapter 10 (CONSCIOUSNESS AND AMBIGUITY OF MEANING) shows how consciousness would be manifested when a meaning is ambiguous. The greater the ambiguity the less the intrinsic meaning and customary consciousness, although extrinsic meaning would be vast.

Chapter 11 (INTRINSIC MEANING, REPORTABILITY AND "SELF CIRCUITS" AS THE KEY REQUIREMENTS FOR CUSTOMARY CONSCIOUSNESS) shows that for customary consciousness to exist there needs to be not only intrinsic meaning and reportability, but also "self" circuits in the brain that reflect the body map and other aspects of self that are hereditary or learned throughout life.

Chapter 12 (THE HIERARCHICAL STRUCTURE OF MEANING) considers that all customary conscious experiences have subcomponents of more elementary meanings from which emerge vision, hearing, taste, smell, touch, etc. These subcomponents are Jonah-minds, which our customary consciousness does not experience. Hence the difficulty in intuitively picturing how consciousness arises.

Chapter 13 (THE INTRINSIC ORIGIN OF THE SENSES) shows why all the senses arise within the brain and are not properties of the outside world.

Chapter 14 (EXPLAINING CLASSIC PROBLEMS IN THE FIELD OF CONSCIOUSNESS) uses the present proposal to explain a number of classic problems in the field of consciousness:

The Binding Problem
The Chinese Room Issue
Split-Brain Experiments
Blindsight
The Idiot Savant
Mary, The Colorblind Physiologist
Reversed Qualia
Novel Qualia
Consciousness of Self
Consciousness of Consciousness
Consciousness—Is It Useful?
Synesthesia
Can Zombies Exist?
Consciousness of Additional Spatial Dimensions
Consciousness of Higher Levels of Meaning
How Mind-expansive Can Consciousness Be?
Seeing with Sound
Can a Computer Be Conscious?

Chapter 15 (THE UNIVERSALITY OF CONSCIOUSNESS) extends to the universe the idea that consciousness is information. Consciousness exists wherever in the universe there is information and does not need the presence of human beings or even life forms.

Chapter 16 (CONSCIOUSNESS IN SPACE AND TIME) points out that since consciousness is information (meaning) and information (meaning) can encompass both space and time, a given moment of consciousness can reflect events occurring across both space and time.

Chapter 17 (MIND AND THE REAL WORLD—MADE OF THE SAME STUFF?) considers that the entire universe may be made of information and hence consciousness. The universality of information (as consciousness) also can provide an insight into how matter, mass, and energy may have first arisen.

Chapter 18 (QUANTUM THEORY AND REALITY) explores the relationships between consciousness and quantum mechanics. Rather than using quantum mechanics to explain consciousness, it may be better to use consciousness to explain quantum mechanics. The concept of ambiguities of meaning as associated with consciousness can be applied to the understanding of nonlocality in quantum mechanics.

Chapter 19 (FREE WILL, GOD, AND THE SOUL) discusses the idea of God as being the "Consciousness of the Universe" and what this would mean in connection with human consciousness. It is speculated that there could be free will decisions that occur within the rules of quantum mechanics.

Chapter 20 (THE FUTURE) points to useful avenues for future research. It also speculates on future social issues that may arise as computers become more complex, to the level of simulating the complexity of human consciousness.

SELECTED READINGS

Aleksander, Igor (2001) *How to Build a Mind: Toward Machines with Imagination,* Columbia University Press.

Avery, Samuel (1995) *The Dimensional Structure of Consciousness,* Comari.

Axelrod, Robert (1984) *The Evolution of Cooperation,* Basic Books.

Axelrod, Robert (1997) *The Complexity of Cooperation,* Princeton University Press.

Baars, Bernard J. (1988) *A Cognitive Theory of Consciousness,* Cambridge University Press.

Baars, Bernard J. (1997) *In the Theater of Consciousness,* Oxford University Press.

Baars, Bernard J., Banks, William P., and Newman, James B. (2003) *Essential Sources in the Scientific Study of Consciousness,* MIT Press.

Baggott, Jim (1992) *The Meaning of Quantum Theory,* Oxford University Press.

Baron-Cohen, Simon and Harrison, John E. (1997) *Synaesthesia,* Blackwell Publishers.

Barrow, John D. (2002) *The Constants of Nature,* Pantheon Books.

Bell, John (1990) *"Against 'Measurement',"* Physics World 3:33.

Black, Ira B. (1994) *Information in the Brain: A Molecular Perspective,* MIT Press.

Blackmore, Susan (2004) *Consciousness: An Introduction,* Oxford University Press.

Blakeslee, Sandra (1992) *"Nerve Cell Rhythm May Be Key to Consciousness,"* Science Times, The New York Times (27 October):C1.

Blakeslee, Sandra (1995) *How The Brain Might Work: A New Theory of Consciousness,"* The New York Times (21 March):C1.

Breuer, Reinhard (1991) *The Anthropic Principle: Man as the Focal Point of Nature,* Birkhauser.

Brodie, Richard (1996) *Virus of the Mind: The New Science of the Meme,* Integral Press.

Bruce, Colin (2004) *Schrodinger's Rabbits,* Joseph Henry Press.

Cairns-Smith, A.G. (1996) *Evolving the Mind: On the Nature of Matter and the Origin of Consciousness,* Cambridge University Press.

Carter, Rita (2002) *Exploring Consciousness,* Univ. of California Press.

Chalmers, David J. (1995a) *"Facing Up to the Problem of Consciousness,"* Journal of Consciousness Studies vol. 2, no. 3, 1995.

Chalmers, David J. (1995b) *Review of* Shadows of the Mind, by Roger Penrose, Scientific American vol. 272:117.

Chalmers, David J. (1996) *The Conscious Mind,* Oxford University Press.

Changeux, Jean-Pierre and Connes, Alain (1995) *Conversations on Mind, Matter, and Mathematics,* Princeton University Press.

Churchland, Patricia S. (2002) *Brain-Wise: Studies in Neurophilosophy,* MIT Press.

Churchland, Patricia S. and Sejnowski, Terrence J. (1993) *The Computational Brain,* MIT Press.

Churchland, Paul M. (1995) *The Engine of Reason, the Seat of the Soul,* MIT Press.

Churchland, Paul M. and Churchland, Patricia S. (1990) *"Could a Machine Think?"* Scientific American vol. 262: 32–27.

Crick, Francis (1994) *The Astonishing Hypothesis,* Charles Scribner's Sons.

Cytowic, Richard E. (2002) *Synesthesia: A Union of the Senses,* MIT Press.

Davies, Paul (1983) *God and the New Physics,* Simon & Schuster.

Davies, Paul (1991) *The Mind of God,* Simon & Schuster.

Dawkins, Richard (1989) *The Selfish Gene,* Oxford University Press.

De Quincey, Christian (2002) *Radical Nature: Rediscovering the Soul of Matter,* Invisible Cities Press.

Dennett, Daniel C. (1991) *Consciousness Explained,* Little, Brown and Co.

Dennett, Daniel C. (1995) *Darwin's Dangerous Idea,* Simon & Schuster.

Dennett, Daniel C. (1996) *Kinds of Minds,* Basic Books.

Edelman, Gerald M. (1992) *Bright Air, Brilliant Fire: On the Matter of the Mind,* Basic Books.

Edelman, Gerald M. (2004) *Wider than the Sky,* Yale University Press.

Edelman, Gerald M. and Tononi, Giulio (2000) *A Universe of Consciousness: How Matter Becomes Imagination,* Basic Books.

Flanagan, Owen (1992) *Consciousness Reconsidered,* MIT Press.

Flanagan, Owen (2002) *The Problem of the Soul,* Basic Books.

Fletcher, Pat (2002) *Seeing with sound: A Journey into Sight.* Paper at Toward a Science of Consciousness meeting, Tucson, AZ, April.

Folger, Tim (2005) *"If an Electron Can Be in Two Places, Why Can't You?"*, Discover, June: 28–35.

Fraser, Alexander C .(1901) *The Works of George Berkeley,* Oxford University Press.

Freedman, David H. (1994) *Brainmakers,* Simon & Schuster.

Gazzaniga, Michael S. (1998) *The Mind's Past,* Univ. of California Press.

Gazzaniga, Michael S., Bogen, Joseph E., and Sperry, Roger W. (1962) *"Some Functional effects of Sectioning the Cerebral Commissures in Man,"* Proc Nat. Acad. Sci., vol. 48, no. 10:1765–1769.

Gelernter, David (1994) *The Muse in the Machine,* The Free Press.

Georges, Thomas, M. (2003) *Digital Soul: Intelligent Machines and Human Values,* Westview Press.

Goldberg, Stephen (1990) *Jonah: The Anatomy of the Soul,* MedMaster, Inc.

Goldberg, Stephen (1996) *The Jonah Principle: The Basis for Human and Machine Consciousness,* MedMaster, Inc.

Goldberg, Stephen (1998) *Consciousness, Information, and Meaning: The Origin of the Mind,* MedMaster Inc.

Goldberg, Stephen (2003) *Clinical Neuroanatomy Made Ridiculously Simple,* MedMaster Inc.

Goldberg, Stephen (2004) *Clinical Biochemistry Made Ridiculously Simple,* MedMaster Inc.

Goldberg, Stephen (2004) *Clinical Physiology Made Ridiculously Simple,* MedMaster Inc.

Goswami, Amit (1993) *The Self-Aware Universe: How Consciousness Creates the Material World,* Penguin Putnam Inc.

Gregory, Richard, L., ed. (1987) *The Oxford Companion to the Mind,* Oxford University Press.

Gribbin, John (1984) *In Search of Schrodinger's Cat: Quantum Physics and Reality,* Bantam Books.

Gribbin, John and Rees, Martin (1989) *Cosmic Coincidences: Dark Matter, Mankind, and Anthropic Cosmology,* Bantam Books.

Harrison, John (2001) *Synaesthesia, the Strangest Thing,* Oxford University Press.

Harth, Erich (1993) *The Creative Loop: How the Brain Makes a Mind,* Addison-Wesley.

Hebb, Donald O. (1954) *"The Problem of Consciousness and Introspection,"* in *Brain Mechanisms and Consciousness,* ed. J.F. Delafresnaye pgs 402–421, Oxford Univ Press.

Hofstadter, Douglas R. (1981) *"A Conversation with Einstein's Brain,"* in Hofstadter, D.R. and Dennett, D.C. *The Mind's I,* Bantam Books.

Hofstadter, Douglas R. and Dennett, Daniel C. (1981) *The Mind's I: Fantasies and Reflections on Self and Soul,* Bantam Books.

Humphrey, Nicholas (2000) *How to Solve the Mind-Body Problem,* Imprint Academic.

Jackson, Frank (1986) *"What Mary Didn't Know,"* J. Philosophy 83; 5 (May): 291–295.

Johnson, George (1995) *Fire in the Mind: Science, Faith, and the Search for Order,* Alfred A. Knopf, Inc.

Julesz, Bela (1971) *Foundations of Cyclopean Perception,* Univ. of Chicago Press.

Kafatos, Menas and Nadeau, Robert (1990) *The Conscious Universe: Part and Whole in Modern Physical Theory,* Springer-Verlag.

Kandel, Eric R., Schwartz, James H., and Jessell, Thomas M. (1995) *Essentials of Neural Science and Behavior,* Appleton & Lange.

Kauffman, Stuart (1995) *At Home in the Universe: The Search for Laws of Self-Organization and Complexity,* Oxford University Press.

Koch, Christof (2004) *The Quest for Consciousness: A Neurobiological Approach,* Roberts and Co.

Kurzweil, Ray (1999) *The Age of Spiritual Machines: When Computers Exceed Human Intelligence,* Penguin Books.

Lederman, Leon (1993) *The God Particle,* Houghton Mifflin Co.

Locke, John (1690) *Essay Concerning Human Understanding,* Basset.

Mansbridge, Jane J. (1990) *Beyond Self-Interest,* Univ. of Chicago Press.

Mass, Wendy (2003) *A Mango-Shaped Space,* Little, Brown, and Co.

McCrone, John (1999) *Going Inside: A Tour Round a Single Moment of Consciousness,* Faber and Faber.

Meijer, Peter B.L. (2002) *"Seeing With Sound for the Blind: Is it vision?,"* Paper at Toward a Science of Consciousness meeting, Tucson, AZ, April. http://www.seeingwithsound.com/voice.htm.

Mermin, N. David (1985) *"Is the Moon There When Nobody Looks?"* Reality and the Quantum Theory, Physics Today, pgs. 38–47, April.

Metzinger, Thomas (1995) *Conscious Experience,* Imprint Academic.

Minsky, Marvin (1985) *The Society of Mind,* Simon & Schuster.

Pagels, Heinz R. (1982) *The Cosmic Code,* Simon & Schuster.

Paul, Gregory S. and Cox, Earl D. *Beyond Humanity: CyberEvolution and Future Minds,* Charles River Media, Inc.

Penrose, Roger (1989) *The Emperor's New Mind: Concerning Computers, Minds, and the Laws of Physics,* Oxford University Press.

Penrose, Roger (1994) *Shadows of the Mind,* Oxford University Press.

Penrose, Roger (1997) *The Large, the Small, and the Human Mind,* Cambridge University Press.

Pierce, John R. (1980) *An Introduction to Information Theory,* Dover.

Restak, Richard M. (1994) *The Modular Brain,* Charles Scribner's Sons.

Rosenthal, David M. (1991) *The Nature of Mind,* Oxford University Press.

Rucker, Rudy (1987) *Mind Tools,* Houghton Mifflin Co.

Rucker, Rudy (1983) *Infinity and the Mind,* Bantam Books.

Schneider, Thomas D. (1995) *Information Theory Primer.* ftp://ftp.ncifcrf.gov/pub/delila/primer.ps

Scott, Alwynn (1995) *Stairway to the Mind.* Copernicus.

Searle, John R. (1990) *"Is the Brain's Mind a Computer Program?"* Scientific American 262:26–31.

Searle, John R. (1992) *The Rediscovery of the Mind,* MIT Press.

Shannon, Claude E. and Weaver, W. (1963) *The Mathematical Theory of Communication,* Univ. of Illinois Press.

Shear, Jonathan (1995–7) *Explaining Consciousness—The 'Hard Problem,'* MIT Press.

Shermer, Michael (2000) *How We Believe: The Search for God in an Age of Science,* W.H. Freeman and Co.

Shermer, Michael (2004) *The Science of Good and Evil,* Times Books.

Shermer, Michael (2004) *"Flying Carpets and Scientific Prayers,"* Scientific American, Nov: 34.

Singh, Simon (1999) *The Code Book: The Science of Secrecy from Ancient Egypt to Quantum Cryptography,* Anchor Books.

Smullyan, Raymond M (1981) *"An Unfortunate Dualist,"* in Hofstadter, D.R. and Dennett, D.C. *The Mind's I,* Bantam Books.

Spitzer, Manfred (1999) *The Mind Within the Net,* MIT Press.

Stapp, Henry P. (1993) *Mind, Matter, and Quantum Mechanics,* Springer Verlag.

Sur, Mirganka and Leamey, Catherine A. (2001) *Development and Plasticity of Cortical Areas and Networks.* Nature Reviews Neuroscience 2: 251–62.

Talbot, Michael (1991) *The Holographic Universe,* Harper Perrenial.

Thuan, Trinh Xuan (1995) *The Secret Melody,* Oxford University Press.

Tipler, Frank J. (1994) *The Physics of Immortality,* Doubleday.

Turing Alan M. (1981) *"Computing Machinery and Intelligence,"* in Hofstadter, D.R. and Dennett, D.C., *The Mind's I,* Bantam Books.

Tye, Michael (1995) *Ten Problems of Consciousness,* MIT Press.

Valiat, Leslie G. (1994) *Circuits of the Mind,* Oxford University Press.